"Lyne Piché and Anton Schweighofer have made an important contribution in developing this workbook for clients concerned or in trouble for their use of sexually explicit materials depicting children, and the clinicians who work with these clients. Drawing on their many years of clinical experience working with these clients, and their solid knowledge of the latest scientific literature, Piché and Schweighofer provide an evidence-based program addressing the most common treatment needs in this population in a sensitive and nuanced manner. Clinicians and clients will greatly benefit from this excellent treatment resource".

Dr. Michael Seto, *Forensic Research Director, University of Ottawa's Institute of Mental Health Research at The Royal, Professor in Psychiatry, University of Ottawa, Canada.*

Working with Offenders who View Online Child Sexual Exploitation Images

This comprehensive workbook addresses the use of illegal online sexual images. Focusing specifically on child sexual exploitation material (CSEM), it offers a clear and professional manual for use with men who use CSEM.

Working with clients who access illegal online images is challenging work. CSEM clients have unique characteristics and treatment needs. Designed around practitioner and client needs, each chapter provides a guide for clinicians and a subsequent set of materials for the client. The workbook covers a range of topics such as motivation for change, relationships, thinking patterns, emotions management, sexuality, computer use, Internet safety and future strategies to ensure both client and community safety. Addressing these issues as well as community accountability helps users of CSEM achieve a satisfying life while avoiding future criminal justice involvement. Through this clearly written and structured workbook, clients are given the resources to help manage problematic thoughts and/or illegal sexual behavior. Offering evidence-based strategies rooted in the authors' clinical experiences, the workbook enables the practitioner and client to work productively together to address the issues that have led to their involvement with illegal sexual images.

This book will be helpful to a range of practitioners including forensic and clinical psychologists, as well as those working in correctional settings, such as probation and prison staff, psychiatrists, social workers, counselors and providers of mental health treatment. It is also designed for anyone who has viewed, or is worried about viewing, sexual images of children.

Lyne Piché is a registered psychologist who has worked in the field of forensic psychology for 25 years. She works in private practice in the province of British Columbia, Canada.

Anton Schweighofer is a registered psychologist who has worked in the field of forensic psychology and addictions for 25 years. He works in private practice in the province of British Columbia, Canada.

Working with Offenders who View Online Child Sexual Exploitation Images

Lyne Piché and Anton Schweighofer

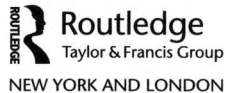

Routledge
Taylor & Francis Group

NEW YORK AND LONDON

Designed cover image: © Getty Images

First published 2023
by Routledge
605 Third Avenue, New York, NY 10158

and by Routledge
4 Park Square, Milton Park, Abingdon, Oxon, OX14 4RN

Routledge is an imprint of the Taylor & Francis Group, an informa business

Library of Congress Cataloging-in-Publication Data
Names: Piché, Lyne, author. | Schweighofer, Anton (Psychologist), author.
Title: Working with offenders who view online child sexual exploitation images / Lyne Piché and Anton Schweighofer.
Description: New York, NY : Routledge, 2023. | Includes bibliographical references and index. | Summary: "This comprehensive workbook addresses the use of illegal online sexual images. Focusing specifically on child sexual exploitation materials (CSEM), it offers a clear and professional manual for use with men who use CSEM"— Provided by publisher.
Identifiers: LCCN 2022059862 (print) | LCCN 2022059863 (ebook) | ISBN 9781032482569 (hardback) | ISBN 9781032478234 (paperback) | ISBN 9781003388142 (ebook)
Subjects: LCSH: Sex offenders—Rehabilitation. | Child sexual abuse—Prevention. | Child pornography. | Online sexual predators.
Classification: LCC RC560.S47 P53 2023 (print) | LCC RC560.S47 (ebook) | DDC 364.15/3—dc23/eng/20230406
LC record available at https://lccn.loc.gov/2022059862
LC ebook record available at https://lccn.loc.gov/2022059863

ISBN: 978-1-032-48256-9 (hbk)
ISBN: 978-1-032-47823-4 (pbk)
ISBN: 978-1-003-38814-2 (ebk)

DOI: 10.4324/9781003388142

Typeset in Minion
by Apex CoVantage, LLC

Access the Support Material: www.routledge.com/9781032478234

Contents

Acknowledgments

Lyne Piché, Ph.D. I would like to thank my family. I could not have done this without your support, patience and care. I love you guys! I would also like to thank my professors, mentors and colleagues over the years. I have enjoyed working with you and I am so very proud of this field of sexual abuse prevention. Finally, I would like to acknowledge my long and fruitful professional collaboration with Anton. We have worked together for so many years that I cannot imagine being in this field without our frequent collaborations, consultations and professional discussions. This book started as a result of our need to better understand these unique clients who appeared following the integration of the Internet into our homes and daily lives. The journey has been interesting and challenging. Thank you for being such an important part of the journey!

Anton Schweighofer, Ph.D. This workbook would not have been possible without the ongoing encouragement and prodding of my co-author, Dr. Lyne Piche. We may squabble over sentence structure and organization, but I am so grateful for you – you are a wonderful friend and colleague. I want to thank Michael Seto, Angela Eke, Kelly Babchishin, Hannah Merdian and the many other researchers who have helped to increase our understanding of men who access child sexual exploitation material (CSEM). Such research provides the necessary guidance for clinicians who endeavor to provide empirically based and effective treatment. Thank you to the many clients who have shared your lives with me and, in so doing, have deepened my understanding of the road to CSEM and how to again find a healthy course in life. Finally, thank you to our publisher, Routledge, for believing in this project.

Introduction

CLINICIAN GUIDE

Working with clients who access child sexual exploitation material (CSEM) is challenging work. Both you and your client are working to address ongoing habits that have been significantly impacting their lives, in many cases, addressing behaviors that have been ongoing for many years. As practitioners, we want to focus on the client's need to motivate themself for change, understand their behavior patterns and help them better manage their behaviors as well as ensure both client and community safety.

It is assumed that clinicians have some expertise in conducting assessments of men who have accessed CSEM. It is also expected that in accordance with the Risk-Needs-Responsivity model, the results of assessments would be used to guide the intensity and focus of treatment. Assessing clients who use CSEM is an area that is changing quickly. It is essential that as a clinician you keep up with the literature in both assessing and treating these clients.

This workbook is based on best practice relating to biological males who have used CSEM. We expect that this workbook would be used with CSEM clients in an individual format or as part of a group setting for CSEM offenders. This workbook is not created specifically for developmentally delayed offenders, brain injured offenders or special-needs offenders. While the concepts may also apply to different client groups, it will be the clinician's responsibility to ensure that the application of these treatment concepts are the best match for your particular client's unique characteristics.

We have designed this workbook to address both the clinician's needs and the client's needs. You will find that the workbook is divided into treatment sections, with a portion dedicated to the clinician and a portion dedicated to the client. The workbook is meant to be followed in chapter order, but you are welcome to find the sections that best address your therapeutic needs. Ultimately, as the treating clinician, you know what will work best for both you and your client. You will need to adapt the materials to the client's individual needs and their particular circumstances. As a registered mental health professional, we encourage you to adapt the information as you see fit. We hope that this workbook will be as helpful for you as it is for the client.

DOI: 10.4324/9781003388142-1

CLIENT WORKBOOK

This workbook is designed to help you stop using child sexual exploitation material (CSEM). We encourage you to use this workbook in conjunction with working with a therapist. This workbook is designed to work in conjunction with an ongoing structured treatment program. Your work with a treatment provider is important to help enhance and deepen your understanding of the concepts discussed in this workbook.

This workbook has a lot of information! The goal of this workbook is to help you better understand your CSEM use and how to address it. If you have any questions about the content of this workbook, discuss it with your treatment provider.

You do not have to read the chapters in order. Some chapters will apply to you while others will not. You may need to re-read the chapters. That is fine. Keep at it and don't give up in your goals for change!

If you are not in a private location or if you do not have privacy in your life, be careful to keep the information in this workbook safe.

We hope that this workbook will be a positive step in your journey to changing your online behaviors.

First Steps

CLINICIAN GUIDE

In your initial sessions with your client, we encourage you to focus on clarifying the treatment process. Clearly outlining the treatment rationale, treatment goals and expected treatment outcomes are important elements of your first sessions. Terminology is also important to clarify. Specifically, you will notice that rather than use the term "child pornography" this workbook uses the term "child sexual exploitation material" or CSEM. In brief, the rationale for this terminology is that CSEM is not simply another type of pornography depicting consenting adults. The term CSEM clearly conveys that such imagery necessarily involves the sexual exploitation of a child, and it is hoped that the use of such terminology will help clients more readily understand the harm that results from the viewing of such images. The term CSEM also allows clinicians to speak to the use of imagery of children that may not be overtly sexual in nature, but which is nevertheless used by clients for sexual gratification.

In addition to ensuring clarity as it relates to the treatment process, treatment goals, terminology and any limitations of confidentiality that you are required to fulfill, we encourage you to clearly define the legal elements involved in online offending. This means reviewing the concept of consent and understanding what is meant by child sexual exploitation material. In also includes explaining the legal definitions related to CSEM use in your jurisdiction. This is also an essential first step. Often clients do not understand the basic elements that comprise the definition of child sexual exploitation material and/or have significantly minimized their use of these images. Exploring the nature of the material, addressing the importance of eliminating these behaviors as well as discussing legal definitions and obvious thinking errors that are observed in your initial sessions can be used to enhance motivation to change.

In addition, assessing for both suicide risk and risk to identifiable children is essential in the initial sessions with your client. While your risk assessment continues throughout your work together, it is important to start by clearly assessing both suicide risk and the risk to any children in your client's environment.

Firstly, ask direct questions to determine if suicide risk is a concern. Many clients who have struggled with their use of child sexual exploitation material or who have recently been detected by the criminal justice system have thoughts about suicide. Suicidal thoughts are quite common for newly detected offenders. Discussing these thoughts openly with your client allows you to monitor risk as well as ensure that your client has a safety plan in place to prevent further harm. Encourage your client to include trusted others as part of their suicide safety plan. Provide your client with emergency contact numbers for local crisis agencies.

DOI: 10.4324/9781003388142-2

Contact additional mental health support services as needed to address any acute mental health requirements. Ensure that you have a suicide prevention plan that is comfortable both for you and for your client.

Secondly, you must evaluate the risk to identifiable children, as this is a fundamental part of our work. Children cannot protect themselves and the ultimate goal of treatment is to keep children safe. Clients are expected to manage their risk in the community and create a team approach with you to help ensure community safety. Talk openly with your client about the children present in their environment and the presence of any urges to offend (both online and contact offenses). Discuss the importance of transparency, openness and honesty throughout the treatment process. Ensure that the client feels safe to disclose any concerns that they may have throughout treatment and clearly define the confidentiality boundaries within a therapeutic relationship. You may need to create an initial safety plan to ensure that the client and the community are safe while you work through program elements with the client. In this case, reach out to relevant community support services for assistance. This may be the inclusion of an accountability partner for your client, the introduction of a CoSA support circle (Circle of Support and Accountability) and reaching out to social services and/or criminal justice partners to help manage any concerns as it relates to your client's risk to the community. Assessing risk, both for the client's safety and for the safety of others in their environment, is an essential first step in treatment.

Assessing the therapeutic alliance is also essential to success. If the fit is not good and the client does not feel comfortable with you as a clinician, refer them to another practitioner with similar expertise. Therapeutic engagement is important for treatment effectiveness and can impact risk management both for the client and the community. Establishing the client's comfort level surrounding disclosure and clearly outlining the need for honesty within the treatment setting are two ways that you can help keep both the client and the community safe. We will talk more about therapeutic alliance and ways to ensure positive feedback between you and the client in more detail in the next chapter.

Finally, as discussed in the introduction, ensure that your treatment plan is based on a solid assessment and applies risk, needs and responsivity principles that are specific to your particular client.

These first steps form the foundation for your work with your clients. Pay attention to the elements that help you successfully set boundaries with your clients and engage them in the process of change. Determine the clients' goals and ensure that these align with your therapeutic expertise and your treatment plan. Start by creating a strong therapeutic alliance as a foundation for your treatment plan.

CLIENT WORKBOOK

Learning Objectives

In this chapter, you will:

a) develop an understanding of the legal definition of child pornography
b) learn why viewing child sexual exploitation material is harmful
c) learn about the topics and issues that will be addressed in this workbook
d) identify whether you are at risk for suicide and what you can do if you are at risk
e) identify if you pose an imminent risk for the sexual abuse of a child and what to do about it

You have taken an important step! You realize something needs to change in regard to your viewing of the sexual images of children. At this point, we want to acknowledge your courage in admitting that there is an issue you want to address. Your decision to engage in treatment may have been triggered by your increasing concern about your viewing of child sexual exploitation material (CSEM), concern raised by someone close to you or perhaps you have been arrested. Whether it is one of these concerns or some combination of these concerns, we are happy to provide you guidance as you begin this journey.

The legal definition of child pornography varies. The following definition from the US federal statute (Section 226 of Title 18) United States Code provides some understanding of how the term can be defined. In the current US federal statute, child pornography is defined as any visual depiction of sexually explicit conduct involving a minor (someone under 18 years of age). Visual depictions include photographs, videos, digital or computer-generated images indistinguishable from an actual minor, and images created, adapted or modified, but appear to depict an identifiable, actual minor.

Of note, a picture of a naked child may constitute illegal child pornography if it is sufficiently sexually suggestive.

In addition, written materials and/or stories of sexual acts involving individuals under the age of 18 also fall under the legal definition of child pornography in some jurisdictions.

We use the term CSEM rather than the term child pornography in this workbook. The term CSEM highlights the reality that a child is being sexually exploited in the very making of such material and again when such material is viewed by adults. This material involves the exploitation of a child. It is also important to consider images of children which are not sexually explicit, but which are viewed for sexual purposes. These images can include photographs of children in bathing suits, in dance class, at nudist sites or in beauty pageant attire. Viewing such images can result in the sexual exploitation of children and the viewing of more clearly sexualized material involving children.

In the following chapters, we will walk with you through a number of issues that are important in helping you to understand how you got to this point in your life. We hope this workbook and your participation in treatment will help you stop viewing CSEM and also help you develop a healthier and happier life. We will discuss factors that can make individuals more vulnerable to viewing CSEM. We will also discuss specific issues related to the role of sex in your life, your sexual interests, whether your viewing of CSEM is part of a larger pattern of problematic sexual behavior and/or is part of a specific sexual interest in children. We will examine and explore the beliefs that helped you rationalize or justify your viewing of CSEM. We will also provide information about the impact on children who are depicted in

CSEM. We invite you to explore what a healthy sex life looks like to you, the nature of your interpersonal relationships, issues related to intimacy and loneliness as well as the development of healthy and sustaining relationships. This workbook will also examine how you manage emotions and unhealthy versus healthy use of the Internet/technology.

For many who find themselves in your situation, thoughts of suicide or self-harm are sometimes present. That is why one of the first issues we want to address is whether you are currently at risk of committing suicide. Even if this is not an issue for you, it may be useful to briefly review the following. This is often a time of turmoil, fear and sometimes hopelessness regarding the future. If you have recently been arrested for the first time in your life, you may be wondering whether you can have a decent life. Will you be able to keep your job? Will people you love and care for reject you? These are common thoughts and concerns. For some, these concerns seem overwhelming and insurmountable. As such, we want to first make sure you are safe.

The following questions can help you take a clearer look at your risk of suicide:

1)	Do you have a history of prior suicidal behavior?	Y	N
2)	Do you suffer from a chronic mental illness?	Y	N
3)	Do you suffer from a chronic physical illness?	Y	N
4)	Have you recently experienced a significant stressor or been arrested?	Y	N
5)	Have you been having thoughts of suicide?	Y	N
6)	Are you feeling hopeless?	Y	N
7)	Are you feeling highly agitated?	Y	N
8)	Have you been engaging in risky behavior?	Y	N
9)	Have you developed a suicide plan?	Y	N
10)	Have you withdrawn from others?	Y	N
11)	Are you actively using alcohol or drugs?	Y	N
12)	Do you have a way to commit suicide?	Y	N

Total # of yes statements _____

If you have answered yes to many or most of these questions, then we highly encourage you to talk to your therapist, call your local crisis line or go directly to your local hospital emergency room. Let someone close to you know what you are thinking so they can support you. Suicide can be seen as a solution to an insurmountable problem but, with help and support, people do get through the strife and turmoil of the moment and find that things get better. Reaching out to others is so very important if you are plagued by suicidal thoughts and impulses to self-harm.

> It is also important to remember that the viewing of CSEM does not mean you are an inherently bad person or are irredeemable. Otherwise good and decent people sometimes find themselves in places they never expected to be. Recovery is possible.

The next issue that we want to address in this chapter is whether your viewing of CSEM has led you to want to sexually touch an actual child. Although a significant percentage of those who view CSEM never touch an child, there are many who have had thoughts of doing so and some who do progress to sexually touching a child or communicating with a child for sexual purposes over the Internet via webcam or in the community. The viewing of

CSEM is a serious act in itself and sexually abusing a child is a criminal act that we want to help you avoid. The costs to the child and to you are simply too great.

If you have been having thoughts and impulses to sexually touch a child and if you have access to children, **you need to take action** to prevent yourself from making matters worse. Although this action may vary depending on your situation, there are a few steps that you should consider. First, if you have easy access to a child and you have been having sexual thoughts about that child, remove yourself from that situation. If this child is your child or your partner's child (a stepchild), you must leave the home and create distance from that child and that relationship immediately. If the child is a relative or friend of the family, find a way to avoid visiting and stop contact with that child. Never be alone with the child. Talk honestly to your therapist about the presence of children in your life. Please confide in a trusted person who can support you and who can help ensure you are not placed in a situation where you might be alone with the child. Even if another trusted adult is present, do not engage in any high-risk behaviors such as bathing the child, swimming with the child, helping the child change their clothes or being in the presence of the child when the child is sleeping.

If you are thinking of sexually touching a child, it is important to ensure that your therapist has expertise in this area, actively apply yourself to treatment and find additional support and help as needed. This may involve some other type of support, for example, the Stop It Now! website, Don't Offend website, B4UAct!, Help Wanted prevention website, Talking For Change website or the Virtuous Pedophiles website. Finding a knowledgeable therapist can be a challenge. Look for guidance through the Association for the Treatment and Prevention of Sexual Abuse (ATSA) website. The ATSA website includes a referral list of therapists throughout the United States, Canada and other countries who are experienced in working with individuals who have had thoughts of sexually touching children. The Safer Society Press also offers a referral service. The National Organization for the Treatment of Abusers (NOTA) in the UK, International Association for the Treatment of Sexual Offenders (IATSO), as well as the Australian and New Zealand Association for the Treatment of Sexual Abuse (ANZATSA) also offer similar resources.

In our experience, some individuals are reluctant to talk to their therapist about sexual thoughts of children or their viewing of CSEM and are concerned that this will require the therapist to report them to authorities. In most jurisdictions, a therapist is not required to report someone who reports they have been viewing CSEM but who has not been sexually communicating or interacting with an identifiable child. In other jurisdictions, therapists are typically only required to report if they believe that a child is at risk of harm. Specific reporting requirements will vary from jurisdiction to jurisdiction and can change over time. Look for a therapist who is experienced in the ethics and legalities of working with clients who have accessed CSEM and clients who report having sexual thoughts of children. It is also important to find a therapist who is emotionally at ease dealing with these issues. Of course, if you have already come to the attention of the criminal justice system for using CSEM, you may already be in a structured treatment program with an experienced therapist.

Questions to consider when working with a therapist include:

1) Is the therapist a licensed helping professional?
2) Does the therapist have experience working with individuals who have accessed CSEM?
3) Does the therapist have experience working with clients who report a sexual interest in children?
4) Does the therapist's consent form include a clear overview of the limits to confidentiality? If not, is the therapist able to provide a clear verbal understanding of their reporting requirements and under what circumstances they are obligated to report and not obligated to report to authorities?

Even if you are not concerned about your risk to an actual child, it is important to work with a knowledgeable therapist to support what you are learning in this workbook. You might recall a time in your life when simply having someone whom you trusted and felt safe confiding in helped you through a tough time. Perhaps it was a close friend, a favorite relative or someone else. Do not underestimate the helpfulness of discussing issues openly with others and the benefits of having a receptive ear. Being in a treatment is an important step toward change.

In the following chapter, we will examine the issue of change.

CHAPTER SUMMARY

- Child sexual exploitation material (CSEM) is the term we employ to identify all material that is used to create sexual arousal with themes involving children. There are many types of legal and illegal images, stories and videos that would be considered CSEM.
- It is illegal to view images, read stories, write stories or otherwise engage in themes that involve individuals under the age of 18 years in sexual scenarios.
- If you are thinking of self-harm, reach out to your treatment provider, local crisis line or hospital emergency department for assistance.
- If a child is at risk and/or if you have thoughts of sexually abusing a child in your community, you must take action to protect that child.
- A mental health professional, as well as a trusted close friend/family member, can be an important source of support in your efforts to change.

Do I Want to Change?

CLINICIAN GUIDE

Facilitating motivation to change is the first step in the treatment process. Motivation is essential in all therapeutic endeavors. We understand that you may be working in a system or an environment that does not encourage the client to structure their own change process. We also understand that you might be feeling limited in the ways that you can create motivation with your clients. There are many ways to improve motivation! Whether it is acknowledged in your treatment setting or not, the choice to change starts and remains with the client.

Focus on motivation to change in your initial sessions. Make it clear that it is the client's decision to change – or not. Explore the pros and cons of change. Discuss theories of change in the context of more general behaviors in order to create a parallel to sexual behaviors. The good life model is one way to help clients visualize their ideal life and start striving toward that life (see Prescott, Willis, & Ward, 2022; Willis, Prescott, & Yates, 2013; Ward & Stewart, 2003 for details). Change will continue to be part of your therapeutic conversation throughout your work with the client.

Change is a process; it can take time and, most importantly, it will likely waver during the change process. Discuss ways that you will address motivation throughout your work together. Discuss how you and the client might address indications that the client's motivation is flagging. We recommend that you include a session feedback form as a strategy to improve communication with your client about their comfort level in sessions and their motivation to apply the skills discussed throughout this workbook. Asking the client to evaluate both their treatment engagement as well as the content of the treatment sessions can help maintain motivation over time. In addition, the GLM fidelity form (see Prescott, Willis, & Ward, 2022) may be another way to assess your therapeutic engagement with the client.

Find creative ways to touch on the topic of motivation throughout your work together. What needs does your client have that you can assist them with in order to enhance their therapeutic alliance? Respect their perceptions related to the change process, communicate openly about their perceptions and seriously consider any feedback that you receive that could improve treatment engagement. As we discussed in Chapter 1, finding ways to enhance and maintain your therapeutic alliance with your client throughout their change process is essential. Whether this includes assisting them to access relevant resources, discussing barriers to change, discussing personalized ways to enhance their coping strategies or recognizing and reinforcing milestones in their behavioral change, these can all work to improve the strength of your therapeutic alliance.

DOI: 10.4324/9781003388142-3

Ensure that the client has the opportunity to discuss how they benefit from accessing CSEM. You may wish to paradoxically ask why someone would want to give up such benefits. Ultimately it should be the client who provides the rationale for forgoing whatever benefits they perceive may have accrued from accessing CSEM. Of course, you can also facilitate discussion of alternative ways that your client can achieve those same benefits. For example, if accessing CSEM is thrilling for your client, this is a benefit and there are alternative ways to create similar sensations. Similarly, if for example your client is using CSEM to manage anxiety regarding sexual performance, the client may well welcome information about alternative approaches to managing performance anxiety. Motivation includes helping your client find their purpose for change. If your client feels that they have already addressed the issues that led to their use of CSEM, you can also focus on their maintenance of the gains they have made and discuss the importance of reviewing treatment themes in order to maintain their changes over time.

If your client is clearly motivated to change but is struggling to stop their CSEM use, it may be timely to introduce the concept of external barriers. As discussed in the workbook section for clients, internal barriers may be enhanced with setting relevant personal goals. In addition, some clients benefit from creating relevant external barriers such as creating a change in their environment to limit their unsupervised use of the Internet. In our experience, clients can benefit from introducing the use of software blockers to provide some initial safety in the beginning stages of treatment. External barriers are discussed further in Chapter 5 Fantasy Management and Chapter 11 Internet Health; however, we encourage you to discuss this option with your client if they are currently continuing to use CSEM.

Staying motivated as a clinician is as important as helping your client find their own motivation. Self-care and professional consultation are two ways to ensure that your motivation remains high throughout your career. There are many ways to ensure your self-care and it is beyond the scope of this workbook to explore them in detail; however, creating a positive balance between your work life and your personal life is an important first step. Creating a self-care routine and maintaining that routine over time is also part of your obligation as a clinician. In addition, clinical consultation is essential to ensure that you are providing the best service to your clients, and also to improve your own work by receiving regular feedback and suggestions from colleagues. If you are unsure where to find a colleague for consultation or a group consultation, you may find services by reaching out to the Association for the Treatment and Prevention of Sexual Abuse (ATSA). ATSA offers resources and the opportunity to communicate with colleagues who specialize in this work. The ATSA website includes a referral list of therapists throughout the United States, Canada and other countries who are experienced in working with individuals who have accessed CSEM and who have paraphilic sexual interests. The Safer Society Press also offers a referral service where you may find a colleague for consultation. In addition, the National Organization for the Treatment of Abusers (NOTA) in the UK, International Association for the Treatment of Sexual Offenders (IATSO), as well as the Australian and New Zealand Association for the Treatment of Sexual Abuse (ANZATSA) also offer similar contact lists of professionals who offer the same specialization.

In many ways, working on motivation with the client is the most important part of this workbook. Make sure that you take the time to engage your client fully in order to set the stage prior to working through the other clinical issues addressed in this workbook.

REFERENCES

Prescott, D. S., Willis, G., & Ward, T. (2022). Monitoring therapist fidelity to the good lives model (GLM). *International Journal of Offender Therapy and Comparative Criminology.* https://doi.org/10.1177/0306624X221086572

Ward, T., & Stewart, C. A. (2003). The treatment of sex offenders: Risk management and good lives. *Professional Psychology: Research and Practice, 34,* 353–360. https://doi.org/10.1037/0735–7028.34.4.353

Willis, G. M., Prescott, D. S., & Yates, P. M. (2013). The good lives model (GLM) in theory and practice. *Sexual Abuse in Australia and New Zealand, 5*(1), 3–9.

CLIENT WORKBOOK

Learning Objectives

In this chapter, you will:

a) consider the benefits you get from viewing CSEM
b) consider the costs of viewing CSEM
c) determine whether you actually want to change your behavior
d) identify what a good life looks like to you
e) identify the barriers to a good life for you
f) identify some personal goals

Costs and Benefits of Problematic Behavior

Changing any behavior can be challenging and it is not uncommon to have mixed feelings about the change process. It is important to acknowledge the benefits one derives from any problematic behavior, whether it is viewing CSEM, problematic alcohol or drug use, gambling or other unhealthy behaviors. People engage in all types of problematic behaviors for complex reasons but there is typically something important that the person gets out of the behavior. You may be thinking, "I don't get anything out of viewing CSEM – only shame and regret". However, if you have been viewing CSEM despite that nagging concern at the back of your mind, despite your understanding that doing so could lead to your arrest or the loss of your relationships, then you have clearly been willing to take some significant risks. When we are willing to take such risks, it is typically because we are getting something out of it. It is important to understand what you are getting from viewing CSEM because unless you have some understanding, you may find it difficult to gather the motivation to change and to make the ongoing commitment to change over the long term. Let's think about what you get from viewing CSEM. Here are some the "benefits" that others in your situation have cited as their reasons for viewing CSEM. Do any of them apply to you and describe your reasons?

. . . .
1   2   3   4   5

1 = Untrue of me
2 = Sometimes true of me
3 = Often true of me
4 = True of me
5 = Very true of me

1) Viewing CSEM helps me escape everyday concerns.	1	2	3	4	5
2) Viewing CSEM is sexually exciting.	1	2	3	4	5
3) Viewing CSEM gives me a sense of power.	1	2	3	4	5
4) Viewing CSEM helps me feel less lonely.	1	2	3	4	5
5) Viewing CSEM helps me feel less bad about the abuse I experienced as a child.	1	2	3	4	5

6) Viewing CSEM helps me express my anger at the world.	1	2	3	4	5
7) Viewing CSEM helps me express my anger at my partner.	1	2	3	4	5
8) Viewing CSEM helps cope with boredom.	1	2	3	4	5
9) Viewing CSEM is a way for me to break taboos.	1	2	3	4	5

If there are reasons that are important to you that are not listed, write them here.

[Other] _____

[Other] _____

If you want to stop viewing CSEM, it will be easier if you are honest with yourself about the benefits you received by viewing CSEM. The issues you may have identified here will help guide you as you begin to figure out what you need to address in your life if you wish to stop viewing CSEM.

Change often starts when you begin to think about how a particular behavior is impacting you. As that process unfolds, some decide to move toward change and others decide to simply keep things as they are. Those who decide they want to change then begin to figure out what they need to do to change and how they can begin to do those things. It may involve changing how you think, how you structure your day, how you deal with feelings and urges, and/or how to involve social supports who will help you change. Of course, even when someone wants to change it can be difficult. Willpower is typically not enough. Concrete action needs to be part of the change process. Change can come slowly, and despite the best of intentions one can slip and fall backward. It takes perseverance and the ability to realize that change is often difficult and full of challenges. Remember that your life will be better as you change; this can be an important motivator and reminder when challenges and setbacks arise.

As you consider the benefits you get from viewing CSEM, it is also helpful to consider the costs. Here are some the "costs" of viewing CSEM that others in your situation have identified; do any of them describe the costs you have experienced?

. . . .
1   2   3   4   5

1   = Untrue of me
2   = Sometimes true of me
3   = Often true of me
4   = True of me
5   = Very true of me

1) Viewing CSEM makes me feel guilty.	1	2	3	4	5
2) Viewing CSEM leads to feeling badly about myself.	1	2	3	4	5
3) Viewing CSEM could end my marriage/relationship.	1	2	3	4	5
4) Viewing CSEM makes me feel anxious afterward.	1	2	3	4	5
5) Viewing CSEM could lead to the loss of my job.	1	2	3	4	5

6) Viewing CSEM could lead/has led to my arrest.	1	2	3	4	5
7) Viewing CSEM could lead/has led people to reject me.	1	2	3	4	5
8) Viewing CSEM has led to online contacts with people I do not respect.	1	2	3	4	5
9) Viewing CSEM has led me to think about sexually touching a child.	1	2	3	4	5

If you have experienced costs that are not listed, write them here.

[Other] _____

[Other] _____

[Other] _____

[Other] _____

By completing these exercises, you have seen that there are both costs and benefits to your behavior. A decision matrix can also help you examine the pros and cons of change. Here is a decision matrix that will help you answer for yourself: What are the benefits of not changing, the benefits of changing, the costs of not changing and the costs of changing your viewing of CSEM?

	Benefits	*Costs*
No Change	*What are the benefits of not changing?* • _____ • _____ • _____ • _____	*What are the costs of not changing?* • _____ • _____ • _____ • _____
Change	*What are the benefits of changing?* • _____ • _____ • _____	*What are the costs of changing?* • _____ • _____ • _____

After considering these questions and after having worked through the decision matrix, where do you stand? What percentage of you wants to stop viewing CSEM, and what percentage of you wants to continue viewing CSEM – whether that is viewing it just occasionally or viewing it more regularly?

_____% of me wants to stop viewing CSEM
_____% of me wants to continue viewing CSEM

If the percentage of you that wants to continue viewing CSEM is less than before, you have taken a step forward! If there is still some percentage of you that wants to continue viewing CSEM, you should understand that such ambivalence is common when people consider changing their behavior. Even if there is some part of you that does not want to change, you can still continue to move forward in therapy and with this workbook. Indeed, as our clients find themselves making progress and feeling happier about the direction of their lives, their motivation often further solidifies and their ambivalence about change lessens.

Seeking a Good Life

It can also be helpful to think about what a good life looks like.[1] By this, we mean what a good life looks like to you specifically. The life that you want may be very different from what others want. So, putting aside the issue of CSEM for the moment, we invite you to consider what your good life looks like for you. You may already be there in many ways, or maybe you are not. In either case, take some time now to write out your ideas and thoughts about what your good life would look like. Be as specific as you can be. For example, rather than saying your good life involves having lots of money, write out some specifics, such as "I want to be able to save $50 every month", "I want to pay all my bills at the end of the month" or "I want to be able to buy a house within five years".

Consider the following areas and provide a specific description of your good life (how you would like your life to look).

1) Your friendships and family relationships

_____

_____

_____

2) Your romantic relationship

_____

_____

_____

3) Your sex life

_____

_____

_____

4) Your emotional well-being

_____

_____

_____

5) Your work

_____

_____

_____

6) Your finances

_____

_____

_____

7) Your physical health

_____

_____

_____

8) Your leisure life

_____

_____

_____

9) Your sense of purpose and meaning in life

_____

_____

_____

Does the life you currently lead match your good life?

___Yes   ___Partially   ___No

If not, why not?

_____

_____

There can be barriers to a good life. Barriers are things that get in the way. Some barriers are internal (e.g. beliefs you hold) and some are external (e.g. racism). Are there things that

have served as a barrier to achieving your good life? Some examples of barriers can include:
(Check all that apply to you.)

1) Difficulty trusting others/suspiciousness/jealousy   ☐
2) Difficulty managing anger and aggressive behavior   ☐
3) A lack of concern about how your behavior impacts others   ☐
4) Problems with ongoing depression or other mental health concerns   ☐
5) Problems with impulsive behavior   ☐
6) Problems managing your sexual thoughts and behavior   ☐
7) A tendency to make poorly considered decisions   ☐
8) Memories and flashbacks and feelings about past traumas   ☐
9) Problems with substance use/gambling   ☐

Sometimes, the barriers to one's good life can overlap with the factors that have made that person more prone to viewing CSEM. For example, low self-esteem and social anxiety can be a barrier to developing a satisfying intimate relationship. It can also sometimes lead people to feel more comfortable viewing CSEM because they find children less threatening and CSEM helps them to avoid facing their fears of developing relationships with adults. This is your opportunity to think about how working to address the barriers to your good life might not only help you stop accessing CSEM but more generally help you achieve the good life you would like to have.

Of the barriers you identified in the prior exercise, which ones would you like to overcome?

1) _____

_____

2) _____

_____

3) _____

_____

5) _____

_____

6) _____

_____

7) _____

_____

What percentage of you wants to overcome the barriers to your good life? _____%

Feel free to revisit these questions because it can take additional time and thought to fully weigh the costs and benefits of making changes in one's life. Consider whether you would benefit from developing social supports who are willing to help you and hold you accountable. Your current treatment provider is a great source of support. If you would like to find additional support, perhaps a community group such as Sex Addicts Anonymous (SAA), Sexaholics Anonymous (SA) or online supports, such as the Virtuous Pedophiles website, would be helpful.

Setting Personal Goals

Setting personal goals can also help. It is important that your goals help you change. It can be tempting to set goals that are too vague or too difficult to achieve. A method for defining goals was developed by Doran (1981) and includes the S.M.A.R.T acronym. According to this model, if you make your goals: Specific, Measurable, Assignable/Attainable, Realistic and Timely, this will help your goals be more effective. For example, rather than saying your goal is never to view CSEM again, start with a specific goal of keeping your computer in an area of your residence where others can view your screen and placing it there by tomorrow at 9:00AM. Of course, you must also consider whether your goal helps you change your CSEM viewing. Another example might be to only use your cellphone in a public place or when someone else is readily able to view your screen. If your screen is readily viewed by others and it will help you change your CSEM viewing behavior, then it is clearly a helpful goal. However, if you live alone, then it clearly is not particularly helpful.

For another example, your goal might be not viewing CSEM for one week starting at 12:00PM today. Are you ready to go without CSEM for a whole week? To help you work toward a healthier and more satisfying life that does not involve CSEM, perhaps your goal is to attend an SAA meeting once a week on Tuesdays and you plan to start next week. Again, that is a helpful goal, but can you get there given your work and family obligations? Do you have a vehicle or is there bus service that will get you there? Would attending SAA be a helpful part of your effort to change your CSEM viewing? Perhaps your initial goal is to read one chapter of this workbook every day at 7:00PM and complete all the associated exercises – starting today. Now that would certainly be a smart goal!

What are your personal goals?

1) _____

_____

2) _____

_____

3) _____

_____

5) _____

_____

6) _____

_____

7) _____

_____

Check and make sure the goals noted here are helpful goals for you. If you are not sure, please talk to your treatment provider.

We hope that what we have reviewed in this chapter helps you make some decisions about viewing of CSEM and, if you do decide to change, we hope you have some added motivation and direction to help you along that path. The first step is to create your goals!

In the next chapter, we will examine the factors that have been found to increase the risk of someone accessing and viewing CSEM.

CHAPTER SUMMARY

- Change begins by considering the costs and benefits of viewing CSEM and the costs and benefits of changing or not changing your behavior.
- Determine what a positive and healthy life looks like to you to foster your motivation to change.
- Determine whether the barriers to the life you want are also issues that have contributed to viewing CSEM.
- Even when we want to change it can be hard and sometimes very frustrating. This is a normal part of the process.
- In the face of the challenges of changing, it can be helpful to find others who will hold you accountable and provide you with emotional and practical support.
- If you determine that you want to change, begin to set some personal goals for yourself!

NOTE

1   We recognize and thank the work of our colleagues Drs. Ward and Stewart amongst others for their work on developing the GLM model of intervention. For more details, see Ward, T., & Stewart, C. A. (2003). The treatment of sex offenders: Risk management and good lives. *Professional Psychology: Research and Practice, 34*, 353–360. https://doi.org/10.1037/0735-7028.34.4.353

REFERENCE

Doran, G. T. (1981). There's a SMART way to write management's goals and objectives. *Management Review, 70*(11), 35–36.

3

The Road to CSEM

CLINICIAN GUIDE

We start this series of sessions with the client's strengths. Prior treatment sessions have focused on safety and the basic elements that required immediate discussion. We now move to enhancing motivation by increasing the client's understanding of their offending patterns, as well as building on their strengths. What are the client's strengths? This is an essential question for you as the clinician. Frequently, clients struggle to identify their strengths. Can you, the clinician, identify your client's strengths? What do they do that works well in their life? What do they know, and how can that knowledge be used to create additional positive change? Can you encourage the client to explore their strengths and add to their own personal understanding of what they can build upon to create a positive life for themselves?

Once you and the client can identify their strengths, focus your clinical attention on increasing your client's knowledge of their behavioral patterns. If your client has had a recent psychological assessment, use this information to structure these sessions. If not, start exploring potential elements that may have impacted risk. You are encouraged to tailor the information in this chapter to the client. Review the longstanding vulnerabilities that relate specifically to the client. Clients are not required to explore all the elements discussed in this chapter, particularly if it is clear that one or more elements do not apply to them.

Allow for an open dialogue in order to discuss the mental health concerns that may be at play in their life. Evaluate personal history as well as family history to identify features that may have been longstanding vulnerabilities for them. For example, these features may be executive functioning difficulties, such as attention deficits which are often genetic, mood disorders or it may be personality features that tend toward self-centered behaviors and/or a lack of concern for others. The particular implications of Autism Spectrum Disorder is explained in greater detail in other sources (see Mahoney, Aygun, & Polen, 2009 for details). Additional information about executive functioning deficits, such as ADHD, and the impact on paraphilias is a burgeoning field (Soldati et al., 2021). Clinicians are encouraged to stay abreast of emerging research.

As a clinician, being well informed about the online environment is essential to ensuring your overall understanding of effective treatment strategies. We encourage you to understand the context of CSEM offending within our understanding of the Internet environment. There is information about the online environment and the impact on CSEM offenders in Chapter 11.

DOI: 10.4324/9781003388142-4

It is essential to complete a thorough assessment to evaluate the client's mental health functioning. Involve local mental health services as needed to secure services offered by community-based mental health providers. Discuss with your client and their physician how longstanding vulnerabilities may be addressed with the use of medications or physical health interventions. Address any obvious mental health conditions that require additional assessment and treatment. If the client is unwilling to pursue additional services to explore identified mental health concerns, work on increasing their understanding of the issues of concern and focus on their motivation to address outstanding problems throughout your treatment sessions.

Once the therapeutic rapport is well engaged, discuss elements particular to the sexual attraction to children. Once your client appears comfortable with your therapeutic approach, it is important to explore these elements in detail. While this theme will be repeated further along in the treatment sessions, an initial discussion about sexual interests, sexual urges and sexual preferences should begin fairly early in the treatment process. Consider the need to implement the sexual urge log as well as implementing external barriers, such as software to block devices accessing sexual and/or violent content, at this time (see Chapter 5 Fantasy Management for more details).

While there are many ways to conceptualize client offending patterns, we encourage you to explore whether your client's behavior was fantasy-driven or contact-driven (Merdian et al., 2018, 2020). Did their use of CSEM include the desire to have sexual contact with children in the community or was their use of CSEM driven by the desire to engage in sexualized fantasy? Another way of exploring this theme is whether the client was using a maladaptive coping strategy or whether the client was facilitating a traditional offending pattern. We encourage you to explore elements related to the offending pathways of CSEM clients and to find a model that best suits your client's needs.

Together with the client, identify a set of risk factors that can help your client better understand and monitor their behavior patterns. Create a plan to identify and address longstanding vulnerabilities that are at play in your client's life. It is not necessary that all longstanding vulnerabilities and triggers be identified at this time. This is an initial discussion and explanation to enhance your client's understanding of their behavioral patterns. Additional focus will be given to this process throughout treatment.

This chapter will help you start creating a template of relevant risk factors. This process assists with creating a useful treatment plan. It also provides the client with some understanding of their offending patterns and behaviors. These initial steps can help solidify motivation and also ensures that the treatment targets are relevant.

REFERENCES

Mahoney, M., Aygun, S., & Polen, M. (2009). *Asperger's syndrome and the criminal law: The special case of child pornography*. www.harringtonmahoney.com/documents

Merdian, H. L., Moghaddam, N., Boer, D. P., Wilson, N., Thakker, J., Curtis, C., & Dawson, D. (2018). Fantasy-driven versus contact-driven users of child sexual exploitation material: Offender classification and implications for their risk assessment. *Sexual Abuse: A Journal of Research and Treatment*, 30(3), 230–253. https://doi.org/10.1177/1079063216641109

Merdian, H. L., Perkins, D. E., Dustagheer, E., & Glorney, E. (2020). Development of a case formulation model for individuals who have viewed, distributed, and/or shared child sexual exploitation material. *International Journal of Offender Therapy and Comparative Criminology*, 64(10–11), 1055–1073. https://doi.org/10.1177/0306624X17748067

Soldati, L., Bianchi-Demicheli, F., Schockaert, P., Köhl, J., Bolmont, M., Hasler, R., & Perroud, N. (2021). Association of ADHD and hypersexuality and paraphilias. *Psychiatry Research*, 295, 113638. https://doi.org/10.1016/j.psychres.2020.113638

CLIENT WORKBOOK

Learning Objectives

In this chapter, you will:

a) Identify your strengths
b) Identify longstanding issues that made you vulnerable to accessing CSEM
c) Identify the differences between different types of CSEM users
d) Identify various problems that might be related to your CSEM use
e) Identify your challenging personality and behavioral styles
f) Identify triggers related to your CSEM use

The clients we work with will often ask, "How did I get here?" It is an excellent question to ask because your understanding of the factors that led you to access and view CSEM can be the key to understanding what you need to address in order to never do so again. Your treatment provider will help you identify the factors that led you to use CSEM. Your self-reflection and honesty will play an important part in this process. We will address this issue in more detail but before we do, we also want to remind you that you have strengths.

Your Strengths

If you have just been arrested or perhaps your spouse has left you as a result of your CSEM use, it may be hard to think about your strengths. Some people may not have even given any thought to what their strengths are, or perhaps they have come to believe they do not have any strengths. It is precisely for these reasons that it is important to spend some time investigating your strengths.

> Benny is starting to work on his CSEM use. He feels like a failure. When he thinks of himself, he thinks: "I am an idiot!", "I'm useless" and "I'm a fuck-up". He wonders if it is worth trying because he'll fail anyway. Benny has always worked hard. He has some friends, and he is always someone that his friends can depend on for help when needed. Generally, people like Benny. Benny has strengths.

A person's strengths often serve as a foundation for working on and surmounting life's problems. Before we reflect on the areas of concern that may have led you to decide to access and view CSEM, please take some time to consider your strengths.

How have you surmounted past difficulties?

_____

_____

_____

What do you do well?

_____

_____

_____

What do other people like or admire about you?

_____

_____

_____

When asked such questions, what comes to mind? If you can't think of any strengths, is there someone who knows you well that you could ask? Strengths can include any number of characteristics. Perhaps you are hardworking, perhaps when you run into difficulties you persevere, perhaps you are self-reflective, perhaps you are able to admit mistakes, perhaps you are loyal to your friends and family, perhaps you are caring, perhaps you are a good problem-solver or perhaps you have good friends and family who help you when difficulties arise. Of course, there are other possible strengths. Take a moment and list your strengths.

1) _____

_____

2) _____

_____

3) _____

_____

5) _____

_____

6) _____

_____

7) _____

_____

8) _____

_____

9) _____

_____

10) _____

_____

11) _____

_____

If you did not identify any strengths or only identified a couple, please ask someone who knows you well what they would add. Others often see our strengths more clearly than we do. It is important to identify your strengths because seeing that you have strengths and abilities is not only encouraging; your strengths are part of the solution to forming a healthier life that does not involve CSEM.

Longstanding Vulnerabilities

The term "longstanding vulnerabilities" refers to the issues that made you vulnerable to accessing and viewing CSEM. Some of these issues may have been present in your life for months or even years prior to your use of CSEM. These can include biological issues, psychological and emotional issues, life experiences, social issues and the environment you inhabit. You may not be aware of what those issues might be or which apply to you. Often, it is only when we review and discuss someone's life history that some of these issues become more apparent. For example, some people have a history of social difficulties. This can include being bullied in school, difficulties with making and keeping peer-aged friends and a general sense of not "fitting in" with peers. This can lead to feeling more accepted by children and generally feeling more comfortable and able to socialize with children. You can see that in this scenario, the connections to viewing CSEM become clearer. Other people have a longstanding history of general pornography use, a history of having had many sexual partners and a willingness to engage in many different varieties of sexual experiences with females and males. A core sexual belief of "if someone walks and talks, I am interested" can be related to future CSEM use, as it may be only a short step to including CSEM in one's sexual life. Another longstanding vulnerability is a sexual attraction to children. Let's look at some examples.

> As a child, Peter had difficulties in school. He had poor grades and would get into fights. While he reported one incident of sexual abuse at the hands of his babysitter, he had only a vague memory of this event. He believed that his parents removed the babysitter from their home, but he was not offered any counseling at that time. He has had prior arrests. He was caught shoplifting as a youth, and he broke windows at a local high school. As an adult, he has had a series of tickets for speeding and he was once arrested for assault. He has a history of using drugs. Peter has worked on and off and makes just enough money to pay for his needs. He has sold drugs at different points in his life to make ends meet. Peter would begin relationships with women easily; however, he was unable to keep them. Eventually, his girlfriends would leave him. Peter had lots of casual sex with women. Over time, Peter began to spend more and more time alone. He would surf the Internet viewing adult pornography. He started looking at many different types of porn, including CSEM. He knew that CSEM was illegal, but he simply continued to view it because he didn't think about the consequences.
>
> Mike has a big family. He is the youngest of four brothers. Growing up, Mike used a lot of porn. He would use porn that involved people his own age. As he got older, he continued to use porn that involved younger people. Mike noticed that he had a sexual interest in kids. He never talked about it. It led to him feeling depressed. Mike went to counseling for his depression, but never talked about his interest in kids. Mike had a hard time forming relationships because he was afraid that people would find out about this interest. He was ashamed and angry. Mike hated his life. He didn't think it was fair and he hated himself.

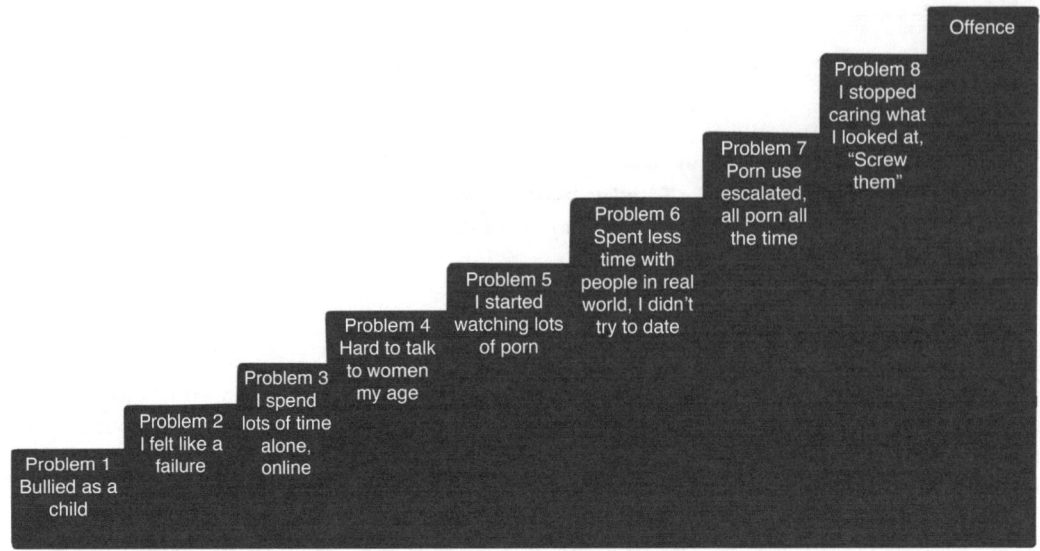

Figure 3.1 Here is an example of how one behavior or one problem can lead to another

Leroy is an older man. He has never been in trouble before. He has just retired. He was a busy professional all his life. Leroy has always had a hard time talking about his feelings. Throughout his life, Leroy would collect stuff – for example, stamps and license plates. Before the Internet, he would watch porn that he collected. He is married. He and his wife would often argue, and Leroy would not tell her about how he was feeling. They stopped having sex over time due to medical reasons. This made Leroy very frustrated. He would ask his wife to have sex, but she would say no. Leroy would manage his frustration by drinking and spending time online. Over time, Leroy began to chat with others online, use online pornography, and view CSEM.

Of course, not everyone with such backgrounds progresses to viewing CSEM. What might be relevant for one person may not be for another. Sometimes one behavior can lead to another. We move from one situation to another, and these situations can increase one's risk of viewing CSEM. Looking for this pattern is sometimes called a chain of events, risk progression, behavioral chain, behavioral progression or staircase to offending, amongst other terms. It is how things go from bad to worse. In this book, we will use the term *behavior patterns*. When you look at the previous examples, you can see how one problem led to another problem, problems that made things worse. When problems start spinning out of control, look for patterns. This often happens when behaviors are connected; your solution to a problem makes you feel worse rather than better and you then create bigger problems instead of solving the initial problem.

Your challenge is to find the factors that made *you* more vulnerable to accessing and viewing CSEM. Here are some issues that can predispose individuals to accessing and viewing CSEM. Check off the ones that you think apply to you.

☐ Feeling lonely
☐ Thinking that you do not fit in with your peers
☐ Thinking that you connect better emotionally with children
☐ A belief that women are rejecting and prone to take advantage of you or are simply not worthy of respect
☐ Difficulties establishing and maintaining stable romantic relationships

☐ A high sex drive, as indicated by the number of sexual partners you have had, a tendency toward impersonal sexual encounters, a high rate of masturbation or frequent time spent consuming adult pornography

☐ A tendency to use sex or sexual fantasy to cope with negative emotions

☐ An interest in varied and unusual sexual experiences (e.g. exposing your genitals to nonconsenting strangers, watching people who are unaware that you are viewing them when they are undressing or having sex, rubbing your genitals against strangers when pressed close together on public transportation or nonconsenting sexual experiences where you or your sexual partner are in pain or are being humiliated)

☐ A sexual interest in children

☐ Conflicted feelings about your own history of having been sexually abused

☐ A tendency to escape into fantasy via video games, second-life games, books or movies

☐ A high rate of general Internet use to deal with boredom, loneliness or other difficult emotions or life events

☐ Using the computer too frequently

☐ A lack of leisure activities

☐ Generally being unhappy with your life

☐ Other

_____

_____

☐ Other

_____

_____

Identifying any of these issues will give you an opportunity to better understand how you eventually made the decision to access and view CSEM. More importantly, you will have a better idea of the issues you will need to address if you are to develop a healthy life that does not include CSEM.

Sexual Attraction to Children

We have already noted that some who access CSEM are sexually attracted to children. Indeed, research suggests that a significant proportion of individuals who access CSEM have an attraction to prepubescent or pubescent children. Pedophilia is the sexual attraction to pre-pubescent children. Hebephilia is the sexual attraction to pubescent children (i.e., children with limited sexual development) typically in the 11- to 14-year-old range. Some individuals are only attracted to prepubescent children. Some individuals are attracted to prepubescent and pubescent children. Some men are attracted to children and adults. Many men struggle to admit pedophilic and/or hebephilic interest, even to themselves. One of the barriers of being honest with yourself and trusted others is the stigma and shame that is associated with a sexual attraction to children. Notably, it may be that some individuals are born with a sexual attraction to children; it is not something that is chosen by them. It is also important to remember that there is a big difference between having such an interest and sexually abusing children. There are men who are sexually attracted to children but who never sexually assault a child. As such, if you have such an interest, it is important to remember that while you may not have chosen to be attracted to children, you do have a choice about how you manage it.

If you have a sexual attraction to children, it is very important that you are honest about that attraction – to yourself and to others who you trust and who can help you.

Generally, those who have a sexual attraction to prepubescent children notice the attraction early in their own sexual maturation. Sometimes they find they are attracted to children their own age but as they get older, they remain attracted to children while their peers develop a sexual interest in sexually developed peers. The attraction to prepubescent children can vary in its intensity but in true cases of pedophilic interest, the interest continues over time. Individuals with pedophilic interest are sexually attracted to prepubescent boys, girls or both. Those individuals who are also sexually attracted to adults may find themselves fantasizing about sex with children when having sex with an adult partner. They may also express their interest by masturbating to thoughts of prepubescent children and by viewing CSEM. Some act out this interest by engaging in a contact offense against a child.

As noted earlier, hebephilia is an enduring sexual interest in pubescent children. As with pedophilia, such an interest likely first becomes noticeable when the individuals are in their teens, and the interest continues to be present over time. Again, those with this interest may be sexually interested in boys, girls or both. Some may also have a sexual interest in adults.

Some individuals are exclusively sexually interested in children, some have an interest in children and adults and some are exclusively sexually interested in adults. On this chart, put a mark on the line to indicate how sexually interested you are in the following age categories (where 0% means you have no interest and 100% means that it is your only sexual interest) and notice whether it is males or females or both to whom you are sexually attracted:

Prepubescent male children (boys without sexual development)

0%   50%   100%

_____

Prepubescent female children (girls without sexual development)

0%   50%   100%

_____

Pubescent male children (boys approximately age 11 to 14)

0%   50%   100%

_____

Pubescent female children (girls approximately age 11 to 14)

0%   50%   100%

_____

Late male teenagers (approximately age 15 to 17)

0%   50%   100%

_____

Late female teenagers (approximately age 15 to 17)

0%   50%   100%

_____

Fully sexually developed men (age 18 and above)

0%	50%	100%

Fully sexually developed women (age 18 and above)

0%	50%	100%

If you have recognized that you have a significant or even partial sexual interest in children, then you have taken an important step. This interest is a very important factor in helping you understand why you accessed CSEM. Moreover, being open about this interest will allow you to put interventions in place that will help you manage your sexual interest. We will discuss how to do this in more depth in the following chapters.

Perhaps you have determined that you are interested in those who are sexually developed but who are about 15 to 17 years of age. While sexual arousal to those who are sexually developed is typical, you will need to work on directing your sexual interest toward those who are of legal age. If you are exclusively interested in fully sexually developed adults, then you will need to examine the other longstanding vulnerabilities that may have contributed to your viewing of CSEM.

Different Types of CSEM Users

Fantasy is an act of the imagination. This may be represented as mental images (e.g. mental movies) or sexual thoughts (for example, "I'd like to have sex with her"). A fantasy can be deliberately brought to mind, or it may simply appear. The nature of the fantasy is reflective of and may perpetuate your interest in children. For some men, the viewing of CSEM can be an end in itself. The viewing of CSEM is motivated by a desire to indulge in sexual fantasies. The viewing of CSEM can also be a desire to indulge in a specific sexual interest in children. Some men have no interest or intention to have actual sexual contact with a child. For others, viewing CSEM is part of a larger motivation to not only view CSEM but to engage in sexual contact with a child.

If an adult's motivation is sexual contact with a child, the viewing of CSEM may be part of a larger belief system that children are inherently sexual beings or that the adult is helping the child learn about sex. Such an adult may not believe that having sex with a child will cause harm. Alternatively, the adult might believe that there could be harm to the child, but that one should be able to do what one wants to do. We call individuals who use CSEM with an intent to sexually offend against a child contact-driven users of CSEM (Merdian et al., 2018)

There are those adults who use CSEM and do not have an interest in sexually offending against a child. The lack of intent to may be because the adult realizes the harm that results from sexual abuse. The individual may also have good self-control. We call individuals who use CSEM and who do not have an interest or an intention to sexually abuse a child fantasy-driven users of CSEM (Merdian et al., 2018)

Your treatment provider may have identified your tendency to be in either one of these categories. To better understand and explore your thoughts about this issue, check any of the following statements that apply to you:

1. ___ My viewing of CSEM was part of a larger pattern of escape into pornography and sexual fantasy of all types.
2. ___ My viewing of CSEM fulfilled my interest in viewing or fantasizing about taboo sexual activities.

3. ___ My viewing of CSEM fulfilled my interest in viewing and sexually fantasizing about children.
4. ___ I believe that sex between an adult and a child does harm to the child.
5. ___ I do not want to do harm to a child.
6. ___ My viewing of CSEM fueled my interest in having sexual contact with a child.
7. ___ I hoped to have online sexual encounters with children.
8. ___ I believe that sex between an adult and a child does not harm a child.
9. ___ I hoped to make online contact with children so that I could develop a relationship with a child.
10. ___ I hoped to make online contact with children so that I could later meet in person and develop a sexual relationship with a child.
11. ___ I believe that sex between an adult and a child is okay and might even help the child in some way.

If you checked statements #1 to #5, then you have the characteristics of a fantasy-driven user of CSEM. If statements #6 to #11 apply to you, then you have characteristics of a contact-driven user of CSEM. Of course, these statements are not the only way explore this issue. It is up you to be honest with yourself about your motivations. An honest discussion is essential if you are to fully come to an understanding of the factors that contributed to your viewing of CSEM. If questions #1 to #5 apply, you will need to focus on issues related to your general coping skills, your tendency to use escapism to cope, your tendency to retreat into sexual fantasy to cope and your possible sexual interest in children. If questions #6 to #11 apply, not only will you need to address the issues noted here, but you will also need to address your beliefs that justify adult and child sexual activity as well as any avenues that might allow you to seek actual contact with a child.

I believe I am more like a fantasy-driven user of CSEM. ___Y ___N
I believe I am more like a contact-driven user of CSEM. ___Y ___N

Problems Related to CSEM Use

This section looks at things that have led others to access and view CSEM. In some cases, we discuss conditions that only professionals with the right training and licenses can properly diagnose. This information is provided here for you to explore and discuss with your treatment provider.

Thinking Too Much About Sex

Do you think about sex to the degree that it distracts you from important issues in your life? Do you think about sex so much that it starts to interfere with tasks that you want to get done? You may be thinking too much about sex if you are having many sexual partners, frequenting prostitutes, attending strip clubs and/or frequently and regularly using legal adult pornography. If you are in a relationship, do you have multiple affairs? Do you masturbate too much? Do you orgasm most days? Frequently thinking about sex, masturbating and/or pornography use over time can become less stimulating. It becomes less exciting. For some people, they will start to seek out more sexually stimulating experiences, both in the real world and/or online. Seeking novelty can be part of the process of accessing CSEM. This tendency to be preoccupied with sex can lead some men to decide to access CSEM and to continue accessing CSEM over time.

Substance Use

Drug and alcohol use is common in our society. A longstanding tendency to use alcohol and/or drugs does not "cause" someone to view CSEM. However, if you have a history of problematic drug and/or alcohol use, you will need to consider whether your drug and/or alcohol use may have made you more vulnerable to unhealthy behaviors, such as the viewing of CSEM.

It will be difficult to make positive changes in your life and to address your CSEM use if you have a substance use problem. We will consider acute intoxication later in this chapter when we examine the triggers that may have contributed to your use of CSEM. Consider the need to address your substance use problem as part of your plan to better manage your CSEM use.

A comment about the abuse of pharmaceutical drugs: You may have a history of abusing prescription drugs. Many people are addicted to prescription drugs and suffer addictive cycles of tolerance and withdrawal. If this is the case for you, address your abuse of prescription drugs in the same vein as drug and alcohol abuse listed here.

While it is beyond this workbook to go into detail about drug and alcohol addiction treatment programs, there are many wonderful programs in the community to assist you with your drug, alcohol or prescription drug abuse. Many programs are available for free. For example, there are community support groups such as AA (Alcoholics Anonymous) or NA (Narcotics Anonymous) or, if you prefer an alternative to 12-step groups, there is SMART (Self-Management and Recovery Training). In addition, there are a host of rehabilitation centers available in many communities that offer both day programs and residential care. Many rehabilitation centers offer both private-pay programs and government-funded care. In some cases, your employer may be able to assist you in covering the cost related to your drug and alcohol treatment program. Talk to your treatment provider about additional resources in your community. As with everything else, the first step is to recognize that you have a problem and then create a plan to address your addictions as part of your desire to avoid any future CSEM use.

Autism Spectrum Disorder

Autism Spectrum Disorder (ASD) is a biologically-based developmental disorder. People with ASD suffer from impairments in their ability to interact with others and their ability to communicate, and they have a restricted range of behaviors or interests. ASD can range in severity from those who are very handicapped by their symptoms to those who are able to function relatively well in society. If your treatment provider has identified concerns related to ASD, it will be important for you to understand what this means.

Difficulties with social interactions are characteristic of ASD. Difficulties with social interactions can be the result of a difficulty viewing the world through the eyes of others. People with ASD can misunderstand other peoples' feelings and intentions and they can be oblivious to what others are feeling. ASD individuals tend to miss social cues and, as a result, will be seen as socially "odd" or inappropriate by others. This in turn can lead to difficulties with building friendships and relationships. Compared to their peers, youths with ASD may seem more naïve and immature. The tendency to hold special interests that are not appropriate for their age, such as an interest by a fifteen-year-old in cartoons or action figures or dinosaurs, can result in further social rejection. As a result, it is not unusual for those with ASD to become "loners". At the same time, because of the desire for social connection and their naiveté, those with ASD can sometimes be taken advantage of by others or be subject to bullying. Such difficulties can leave those with ASD feeling lonely and discouraged about the possibility of building relationships with peers. This can be a potential step toward seeking out unhealthy or inappropriate activities, such as CSEM, to cope with loneliness. Those with ASD can also struggle to understand whether behaviors such as making very blunt or hurtful comments to friends are socially appropriate. This difficulty with understanding social norms and the feelings of others can leave those with ASD struggling to understand what is wrong with viewing CSEM. An additional characteristic of those with ASD is a tendency to become intensely absorbed in activities, behaviors and interests. This tendency to become obsessed with a particular interest can, of course, also extend to the Internet and sexual matters – including CSEM.

> Tyrell has a long history of collecting things. His room is always immaculate and very organized. He started collecting the lids of jars as a kid. He moved on to collecting stamps, coins and historical work-related badges. Tyrell started spending time online and found that there were people interested in CSEM images. He started to collect these images, and he spent hours and hours organizing and categorizing these images. Tyrell didn't really see the problem in his behavior. He didn't see why other people might be upset by his collection. He became obsessively absorbed in the collection until the police came to arrest him. He told police he was surprised that this behavior would be a problem to others.

Difficulties with Attention and/or Hyperactivity

Some individuals suffer from a lifelong difficulty with attention and/or hyperactivity. Attention Deficit Hyperactivity Disorder or ADHD is, like ASD, a developmental disorder. The presence of ADHD is often first identified when children begin to attend school but, particularly for those who are more inattentive than hyperactive, the issue is sometimes not identified. This can make it very difficult for children suffering from ADHD as they can struggle with schoolwork and social relationships. Over time, this can compound and contribute to low self-esteem, frustration, aggressive behavior and impulsive breaking of rules. Individuals with ADHD also tend to be at increased risk for the development of problematic alcohol and/or drug use. As with ASD, the presence of ADHD does not "cause" someone to view CSEM. However, such traits could make someone more vulnerable to social difficulties and impulsive behavior. This, along with other factors, can make someone more vulnerable to accessing CSEM and may make it difficult to cease using CSEM.

ADHD is an important treatment consideration not only because of the role it may play in making someone more vulnerable to accessing CSEM but because, if present, it can also significantly interfere with the ability to focus and apply oneself to CSEM-specific treatment. If your treatment provider has identified this as a concern for you, consult with a mental health professional with a specialty in attention disorders or a physician for additional assistance. Fortunately, ADHD can be addressed through cognitive behavioral treatment and pharmacological treatment.

Depressed Mood

Everyone feels sad sometimes, and having a depressed mood is not necessarily the same thing as suffering from clinical depression. Clinical depression is more intense, longstanding and debilitating than simply a low mood. When you are suffering from depression, you cannot just shake it off. The feelings don't simply go away. Depression can start before a person decides to access CSEM, or it can sometimes follow from the self-criticism and self-loathing that occurs as someone struggles with their involvement with CSEM. In some cases, depression occurs following an arrest for accessing CSEM and the cascade of stressors and feared outcomes after such an event. Whether depression started before your use of CSEM, occurs at the same time as viewing CSEM, or follows a related arrest, it is important to deal with it. Determining whether you suffer from depression is complicated. If your treatment provider has identified this as a concern, it will be important to consult with a mental health professional and/or your family doctor for further assistance.

Anxiety

Anxiety can come in various forms. Worry is often an indicator that anxiety is a problem for you. How much do you worry? What do you worry about? Like depressed mood, anxiety can occur before the use of CSEM, it can start as a result of viewing CSEM or it can result from the consequences of an arrest for viewing CSEM. Sometimes, CSEM is used to cope with anxiety. Spending time online can keep you from addressing your anxiety. If you experience intense, excessive and persistent worry and fear that interfere with your ability to function, it is important that you deal with this problem. If your treatment provider has identified this as a concern for you, it is important to talk to a mental health professional or your family doctor about your concerns. Anxiety can impact all aspects of your life. Don't ignore your concerns about anxiety!

Personality and Behavioral Styles that May Hamper Change

Some personality and behavioral styles may hamper your efforts in changing your CSEM use. We all have strengths and weaknesses. The trick is to find solutions to your particular challenges. Review the information presented here to see if some of it might be helpful to you.

Thrill-Seeking

Thrill-seekers are folks who really like experiencing an adrenaline rush. Life goes too slowly, so you need to crank it up! Finding that rush is important and becomes an essential part of your day. Activities that get your blood boiling, your heart racing and maybe even give you that sensation of having tunnel vision for a moment are thrill-seeking activities. Making life exciting may be very important for you. You may be the type of person who hates this feeling or, alternatively, you might be the type of person who loves it! People who are thrill-seekers are often told to tone it down, calm down and stop taking risks. That advice is often unhelpful, as it can feel like criticism, it can be difficult advice to follow or it simply does not fit with the type of life that you want to lead. It can push you to start seeking thrills that are secretive and unknown to your friends and family, who may not understand or respect your personality style. As you can imagine, engaging in secret thrill-seeking behaviors can propel you to CSEM use.

Thrill-seeking behaviors can lead to problems. These behaviors give you a thrill but can result in negative consequences to yourself or others. Some examples are affairs, risky "hook-ups", speeding on public roads, overspending, and taking risks that endanger your physical health or bystanders' physical health.

Not all thrill-seeking necessarily results in negative consequences. Positive thrill-seeking activities provide an adrenaline rush but also allow you and others around you to be safe. Examples of positive thrill-seeking activities would be rock climbing, extreme sports, car racing at the local racetrack, sky diving, scuba diving, off-road ATV, mountain biking and any sport or activity that allows you to push your limits in a legal way. If you are a thrill-seeker, finding positive thrill-seeking activities will be an important part of your safety plan to manage your CSEM use.

Answer the following questions by putting a mark on the line where you fall (0% = not at all and 100% = absolutely)

Am I a thrill-seeker?

0%   50%   100%

_____

Do I enjoy adrenaline, excitement and/or do I like things that go fast?

0%   50%   100%

_____

What does being a thrill-seeker mean to me?

_____

_____

_____

_____

_____

What negative thrill-seeking activities have I tried in the past and what were the consequences to me and others?

_____

_____

_____

_____

_____

What positive thrill-seeking activities have I used in the past?

_____

_____

_____

What positive thrill-seeking activities am I willing to try now?

_____

_____

_____

If you used to be a thrill-seeker but cannot do so due to physical health problems or limitations, it will be very important for you to find an alternative thrill-seeking activity that is not online. Perhaps you will want to try getting involved in competitive card playing, games groups, debate groups, model building/engineering projects, darts or any other non-strenuous thrill-seeking activity. It is possible to engage in thrill-seeking activities that are not based solely on your physical fitness.

Rule Breaking

Sometimes people really like to break rules, dislike authority or don't like to take advice or direction from others. People who don't like rules tend to break them out of principle, for the fun of it or to see if they can get away with it. If you have such tendencies, your needs will come first, before the needs of others in your life and in your community. How do you consider the needs of others along with your own needs? Do the needs of society as a whole have a place in your decision-making? If not, then you may well be exhibiting what are termed antisocial tendencies.

Having antisocial tendencies can challenge your ability to work cooperatively with others. Cooperation is essential to achieving interpersonal goals. We focus on cooperation to ensure that our needs and other people's needs are respected. If you happen to have antisocial tendencies, you may have known that using child sexual exploitation material was illegal but didn't care about that fact or the consequences associated with that decision. If this sounds familiar to you, it will be important for you to find clear, specific and personal reasons why it is in your best interests to follow the rules and not break the law. This will help you make better choices. Why would it be in your best interests to engage in legal behaviors? Carefully consider and notice when you are telling yourself things that allow you to break the rules, such as "It doesn't matter", "Fuck them", "I can do what I want" and "It's a stupid rule". We will explore the attitudes and beliefs supporting CSEM use in a later chapter. The importance of managing your unhelpful thoughts will go a long way to helping you make better decisions both for yourself and for others.

If you are a rule breaker, stop for a moment to reflect on the impact of your antisocial tendencies.

Breaking the rules has cost me:

_____

_____

_____

The advantages of following the rules in the future include:

_____

_____

_____

If you continue to struggle with these tendencies, talk to your treatment provider for assistance.

Passivity

Being passive means that you do not address obvious problems and do not set boundaries or reasonable limits in your relationships with others. You might believe that you are powerless to change what happens in your life. This lack of agency – "I can't", "It never works", "They don't listen to me" – can keep you stuck in a negative loop of unhelpful behaviors. Being passive means not taking charge of your life. Can you direct your life? Feeling like you can't change key aspects of your life can cause problems. Assertiveness is an important skill.

At times, when people who are passive attempt to become assertive, they overshoot and behave in aggressive ways. Notice if you tend to be aggressive rather than assertive. Alternatively, some people move from being aggressive to passive but struggle with finding the balance of being assertive. Being assertive, rather than aggressive, is the healthy middle ground. If passivity is a problem for you, ask yourself:

What do I want?
What do I need?
How can I communicate my needs and wants productively to others?

These questions can set the stage for you to become assertive in your interactions with others. You can change your environment. You can change your life to suit your needs. This takes thought and perseverance. Addressing a passive interpersonal style is possible. Seeking the assistance of a mental health professional in your community can help you further address these concerns. You may also find resources to assist you with this problem in the Recommended Readings section of this workbook.

Obsessive-Compulsive Behaviors

As noted earlier, there are those on the autism spectrum who can become intensely engrossed in activities and behaviors. However, even if one is not on the autism spectrum, there are indications that those with obsessive thinking patterns and compulsive behaviors may be more prone to problematic Internet use. Symptoms can range in severity. Individuals with such tendencies may find these thoughts and behaviors upsetting and distressing, or they may simply view them as part of who they are as a person. If these types of behaviors are undermining your functioning, your relationships and, particularly, if they played a role in your desire to collect, retain and organize CSEM, then you will benefit from finding methods to better manage and cope with them. Talk to your treatment provider about how to manage anxiety and obsessive-compulsive behavior.

Unhealthy Relationship with the Online Environment

When thinking about issues that may have made you more vulnerable to accessing and viewing CSEM, it is necessary to consider the online environment and your relationship with the online world. The advent of the Internet has brought many positives: increased and easy access to information, improved ability to communicate with others, both in writing and with face-to-face video, and the opportunity to be immediately and continuously be entertained and distracted in countless ways. However, the Internet can also lend itself to the development of problematic behaviors.

For those who are lonely, depressed, or anxious, the Internet can be an attractive refuge from the daily difficulties of life. It can be easier to spend hours on the Internet rather than work on improving your social skills or face your feelings of loneliness. The fact that access to such a refuge is just a click away makes it harder to resist! Perhaps long before you accessed CSEM, you were already finding that your use of the Internet was problematic. Perhaps you found yourself spending time online when you needed to be sleeping. Perhaps others in your life complained about the amount of time you were spending online. Perhaps you regularly blocked out disturbing thoughts about your life by thinking about using the Internet or going online, or perhaps you turned down invitations from others so that you could go online instead. If any of this sounds familiar, you will need to consider how your general use of the Internet made you vulnerable to accessing CSEM. Examining your Internet use also means thinking about what you will need to do in the future if you are to avoid such issues.

The Internet can provide a false sense of intimacy. Communicating with others online from all parts of the world can bring a sense of being known, liked and even respected by others. You may perhaps have a sense that your online social contacts are easier to talk to; that it's easier to share information with people you contact online than with people you see in the offline world. You may find that you develop a sense of emotional closeness to your online social contacts. For those who have struggled with social relationships and who have struggled to feel close to others, this can be an intoxicating experience. The Internet becomes a way to meet your emotional needs. Unfortunately, these online relationships likely lack the real trust, transparency and mutual vulnerability that is the stuff of true intimacy. The search for intimacy can make Internet users vulnerable to immersion in an online world. It also puts you at risk of developing a problem with your online behaviors.

When using the Internet, there is often a false sense of anonymity. Perhaps there were occasions when you found yourself more willing to view "politically incorrect" websites, adult pornography or CSEM because you held the belief that no one would know. Of course, the Internet is not anonymous. The places we visit online leave traces and can be tracked back to us. The problem is that when you are sitting alone late at night, it is easy to believe that "no one will know". The ability to ignore the fact that your actions are not anonymous makes it much easier to step over the line – a line that you would not have stepped over if you had been able to see and acknowledge that your actions were not anonymous.

When we view images on the Internet, it is also easier to emotionally distance ourselves from our actions and the implications of our actions. It is for this reason that people make hurtful and malicious online comments to other people they do not even know—comments they would never make in a direct face-to-face interaction. When it comes to viewing CSEM, this aspect of the Internet experience can make it easier to lose sight of the reality that the children in CSEM are being sexually exploited and abused. There can be a sense that those children are simply images on a computer screen; they are somehow not real and are not actually being harmed. In some cases, the children depicted are clearly from other cultures and other parts of the world, and this also can lead you to see the children as somehow being less real.

If the Internet problems outlined here seem familiar, you will need to understand the impact of the online environment on your offending pattern. Remember that what you view on the Internet can have real-world implications. Real people and real children are adversely impacted by what you do online.

Consider if the following apply to you (check all that apply):

1. ___ I have tended to spend too much time online.
2. ___ I have coped with difficult feelings by retreating to the Internet.
3. ___ I have developed online relationships with strangers and came to believe that they were important supports or came to feel emotionally close to them.

4. ___ Because I felt anonymous online, I was more willing to look at sites I would not have looked at otherwise.
5. ___ I have viewed the children in CSEM as being less real or not real.
6. ___ I did not see my actions as being harmful.
7. ___ I believe that the online environment is not real.

If any of these apply to you, it will be important to develop a plan with your treatment provider for how to have a healthy relationship with the Internet and technology. We will explore the elements of a good plan in upcoming chapters.

Triggers

The term *triggers* refers to thoughts, feelings, behaviors or situations that may have activated your underlying longstanding vulnerabilities so that you actually decided to access CSEM. You may have been lonely, isolated and viewing adult pornography for many years before you finally decided to access and view CSEM. Perhaps there was an important loss or a significant stressor in your life. Or maybe drug or alcohol use started to become a bigger problem prior to actually using CSEM. Perhaps your thinking shifted, and you found yourself thinking that you would not get caught. Maybe you decided that viewing CSEM was a way to prevent you from acting on your sexual interest in children. Or perhaps, after inadvertently being exposed to a sexual image of a child, you decided that the children in the images enjoyed what was being done to them and were not being harmed. Can you recall what was going on in your life *immediately* prior to your decision to access CSEM? Understanding the factors that triggered your involvement with CSEM will help you create an effective plan for change.

In the following exercise, please look at what was happening for you right before you chose to use CSEM. Consider what was happening approximately 24 hours to a week prior to your use of CSEM.

Describe what was happening in your life in that time span:

1. Situational Changes (e.g., job loss, loss of an important relationship, increased problems in your marriage, increased work demands)

_____

_____

_____

_____

2. Changes in Emotions (e.g. increased sadness, loneliness, anxiety, anger, increased sexual urges)

_____

_____

_____

_____

3. Changes in Thinking (e.g., thinking that viewing CSEM is less harmful than acting on your sexual interest in children, thinking that you will not get caught, thinking that the children in CSEM are not harmed, increased sexual fantasy of children, thinking that you should be able to do what you want)

_____

_____

_____

_____

4. Behavioral Changes (e.g., heavier drug or alcohol use, increased social withdrawal, increased time spent browsing the Internet, the purchase of a new computer)

_____

_____

_____

_____

The issues that you have identified here are part of the answer to the question "How did I get here?" These are the issues that you need to address so that you do not find yourself here again. Fortunately, you have strengths, and you will develop new strengths that will help you find a healthier road for your life. Review your strengths, your longstanding vulnerabilities and the triggers that contributed to your decision to access and view CSEM. Use these to help guide you through the following chapters.

My strengths include:

1. _____

2. _____

3. _____

4. _____

5. _____

6. _____

7. _____

8. _____

My longstanding vulnerabilities include:

1. _____

2. _____

3. _____

4. _____

5. _____

6. _____

7. _____

8. _____

My triggers include:

1. _____

2. _____

3. _____

4. _____

5. _____

6. _____

7. _____

8. _____

You will use this information as a guide to working through the upcoming chapters.

CHAPTER SUMMARY

- We all have strengths! Remember your strengths.
- Longstanding vulnerabilities predisposed you to viewing CSEM. Identify your longstanding vulnerabilities and ensure you discuss these with your treatment provider.
- Find positive ways to express your personality style.
- Identify triggers: the thoughts, feelings, behaviors and situations that precipitated your decision to access and view CSEM.

REFERENCE

Merdian, H. L., Moghaddam, N., Boer, D. P., Wilson, N., Thakker, J., Curtis, C., & Dawson, D. (2018). Fantasy-driven versus contact-driven users of child sexual exploitation material: Offender classification and implications for their risk assessment. Sexual Abuse: A Journal of Research and Treatment, 30(3), 230–253. https://doi.org/10.1177/1079063216641109

4

Treatment Approaches

CLINICIAN GUIDE

Most criminal justice treatments utilize cognitive behavioral therapy (CBT). We assume that you have a solid understanding of the concepts related to CBT, as well as the knowledge of how to apply these skills. As a clinician, we encourage you to teach basic CBT skills that will enhance cognitive and emotional awareness and foster change in various aspects of the client's life.

The goal is to start by applying CBT concepts to the client's general behaviors before moving to sexual-specific behaviors. Start by ensuring that the client has basic skills to address their emotions, thoughts and behaviors. We start this section of treatment by increasing the client's understanding of the cognitive elements that relate to their offending. Understanding thinking patterns, unhelpful thoughts and thinking errors are a great way to help clients manage their thoughts and ultimately their behaviors (Beck, 1963). This section continues to focus on improving motivation by helping clients begin to understand and address the beliefs that kept them in their offending patterns. Note that in this chapter, the emphasis is to understand and challenge their ***general*** thinking errors. The goal is to help the client apply these skills in more general areas of their lives first, before addressing more specific thinking errors related to their sexuality and their offending. We will come back to thinking errors specifically related to offending in later chapters of this workbook.

As we explore how to identify and manage unhelpful thoughts, it can be useful to refer to common everyday challenges, such as driving, to help clarify and illustrate the concept of thinking errors. You may wish to draw on your knowledge of the client's specific life circumstances to find examples that engage your client. It is useful to ask clients to identify slightly stressful situations in their lives in order to mine their examples for any underlying thinking errors.

In addition, we encourage the exploration of behavioral strategies to address emotion management. These strategies may enhance the client's ability to cope with negative emotions and better manage problematic behaviors. In addition to some of the suggestions that we offer in the client workbook, we encourage you to explore other behavioral interventions that may be helpful to your client. Exploring grounding strategies, different types of physical activity, mindfulness or other behavioral strategies can enhance the interventions discussed in the client section of this workbook.

In this chapter, we also lay the foundation for the possible need for pharmacological interventions should the CBT approach not be sufficiently effective to curb their urges to use

DOI: 10.4324/9781003388142-5

CSEM. Clinicians are encouraged to ensure that these subjects are discussed from a neutral, educational perspective. Care should be taken to ensure that clients do not feel threatened or intimidated by discussions involving pharmacological interventions to address their risk. Creating hope for change by explaining that there are other available options should the CBT principles not resolve their concerns is the preferred presentation of this information.

Dialectical behavioral therapy (DBT) skills may also be a useful resource for your clients, particularly if they are significantly struggling with emotions management. Your client may also enjoy participating in local CBT and/or DBT groups offered by mental health services to learn and practice additional emotions management skills that could be useful to them. We encourage you to get to know local resources that offer relaxation groups, mindfulness practices as well as emotions management skills. In addition, there are many online support services as well as various apps that can be used by clients to help them improve their general CBT skills. Presenting this information in a variety of ways, for example through additional mental health services, online courses, examples taken from movies or the media as well as using technology (e.g. apps) can help teach effective strategies to manage emotions, thoughts and behaviors.

Overall, this chapter involves teaching the basic skills that are the foundation of your work as a mental health professional. Your approach in this chapter should reflect your usual practice as it relates to teaching basic approaches to behavioral and cognitive change.

CLIENT WORKBOOK

Learning Objectives

In this chapter, you will:

a) Learn the basic principles of cognitive behavioral therapy (CBT)
b) Identify common thinking errors
c) Identify specific behaviors that you can use to help you manage your emotions
d) Consider whether medication may be helpful to you

In the previous chapter, you explored and identified the factors that contributed to your decision to access and view CSEM. The next step involves improving your understanding of how you can begin to address and manage those issues. In this chapter, we will discuss some of the basics of what is called cognitive behavioral therapy (CBT). CBT is used to help you address and better manage strong feelings and reactions. This is one way to help you cope with life in a healthier way. We will also discuss pharmacological treatments so you can better understand what is available and work with your treatment provider to find the approach that fits you best.

Managing Your Thinking

Cognitive behavioral therapy (CBT) is an approach that addresses how a person's thoughts and beliefs influence emotions and behavior. CBT teaches how to manage your thinking so that you have greater control over your emotions and behaviors. The term "cognitive" is simply a fancy word that refers to your thinking. Our way of interpreting the world around us can be influenced by experiences that date back to our childhood and also by our "here and now" thoughts about a specific situation. We always have the ability to manage and change our thinking – even longstanding and ingrained ways of thinking. CBT also addresses how to change your behavior, and we will talk about that in more detail later in this chapter.

It is important to remember that we do not always have the ability to change events outside of ourselves. Even in cases where we can, it may not be wise to try to do so. Indeed, some people get into a lot of trouble by trying to change the behavior or actions of others in an attempt to change how they feel emotionally. We sometimes see this when someone decides they will "teach" another driver how they "should" be driving by tailgating the other driver or by cutting in front of them. Or perhaps someone tends to yell or scream at others to try and force the other person to change their behavior. Such actions can often contribute to further problems. And of course, there are situations that simply cannot be changed, for example, the reality of being arrested or the reality of losing a job. In such situations, the strongest ally we have to help us cope is managing our own thoughts and perceptions. Another way to look at this is by referring to a well-known saying that reminds us that we cannot change the wind, but we can change the direction of our sails. There are occasions where it may be useful to try and address a problematic situation, but you will likely be more successful if you are first able to address your own problematic thoughts and emotions. It is also important to remember that we are not simply talking about "positive thinking" or just wishing for the best. it is about trying to think as rationally as you can. Let's look first at some of the basics of managing your thinking before looking at behavioral interventions.

Managing Your Thinking: The Basics

You may have noticed that the same event can happen to two people, but each person has a different emotional reaction. Perhaps you have been driving with a friend when the car in front of yours does not move forward when the light turns green. Your friend begins yelling and cursing while you remain calm. Why the different reaction?

> Kyle is sitting at a stoplight. His friend Michelle is also in the car. When the light changes, the car in front does not move. Kyle gets angry and starts to yell. Michelle calmly waits. Eventually the car in front starts moving. Kyle thinks, "That shit, what a stupid guy! Damn him! Jackass! If I miss this light, I'm screwed". Michelle thinks, "Oh well, it's not a big deal, I'm glad that we are moving now".

The different reaction is because your friend is thinking about the situation differently than you. Your friend may be thinking that the guy in front of you is deliberately trying to mess up his day, that he might now miss the green light and how that would be terrible. In contrast, perhaps you are simply thinking it is not a big deal if you don't start moving right away. This highlights one of the basic points of managing your thinking – how you think about a situation has more influence on your emotions than the event itself. This example helps illustrate that thoughts and feelings are linked. If you are angry, you have the types of thoughts that lead to anger. If you are anxious, you have the types of thoughts that lead to anxiety. If you have an urge to drink or to access CSEM, it is because you have thoughts that contribute to those urges. These are important points because it means that to use CBT to your advantage, you need to start paying attention to your thoughts. Although that sounds easy, it can actually be quite challenging and it takes practice.

Let's be clear on the differences between an event/situation, a thought, an emotion and a behavior. You need to understand these differences so that you focus on your thinking and managing your thinking in order to manage your emotions and behavior. So let's make sure you understand how to distinguish between an event/situation, a thought, an emotion and a behavior.

An Event/Situation

An event/situation is something that happens externally to you. Generally, this is something you observed (saw, heard, touched, smelled or tasted). In the earlier example, the event was the car in front of yours not moving forward when the light changed.

Thoughts/Self Talk

Thoughts/self talk are what you thought or said to yourself about the event – the inner dialogue that went on in your head. This is often referred to as "self talk". Thoughts typically involve a string of words. These also include attitudes and beliefs. In the earlier example, one of the thoughts was, "If I miss this light, I'm screwed".

Feelings

Feelings are your emotions or what's happening in your body. Emotions can generally be described in one word, e.g., angry, sad, excited or nervous. While this seems straightforward, sometimes people use the word "feeling" to describe what they are actually thinking. For example, when someone says, "I feel like he does not like me", they are actually describing a thought. If you had such a thought, how would you likely feel? Feelings and thoughts are closely related. In this case, there may be other thoughts that need to be identified in order to determine how the person might feel. Is he thinking that he is worthless if the other person does not like him, or does he think the other person's opinion really does not matter to him? If he thinks that it would mean he is worthless, then he will likely feel sad or perhaps anxious. If he thinks the other person's opinion about him does not really matter, then he might feel at ease. This illustrates that you sometimes have to "peel the onion" or dig deep to determine all of the thoughts you are having in order to identify the key thoughts that are impacting your emotions. In the example given, Kyle is feeling angry.

Behavior

Behavior is what you did (including what you said out loud). In our example, Kyle's behavior included yelling and cursing. Sometimes people try and manage their feelings by changing their behavior rather than changing their thinking. For example, they may go for a walk or have a drink. These behaviors may indeed help you get through the moment, but if you do not change how you think about the situation it is likely that problematic feelings will return.

The next challenge is to determine if the thoughts you are having are what therapists refer to as "thinking errors". Thinking errors are unhelpful thoughts. It is important to identify your thinking errors, because such errors can lead to difficulties managing emotions and behaviors that cause harm to yourself and/or others. To identify whether you have a thinking error, you need to ask yourself whether the thought you are having is *a fact or an opinion*. Another way to do this is to ask yourself if there *is little or no evidence* for your thought. The goal is to identify and replace your thinking errors, but you first have to figure out if the thought(s) you are having is a thinking error. From the car example noted earlier, which of the following are thinking errors? Why do you think the thought is or is not a thinking error?

1) That guy is deliberately trying to mess up my day.

   _____

   _____

   _____

   _____

2) I might miss this light and have to wait until the next one.

   _____

   _____

   _____

   _____

3) If I miss this light and have to wait until the next one, it would be terrible.

   _____

   _____

   _____

   _____

Regarding the first thought noted here: can you think of some other reasons why someone might not immediately move forward when the light changes to green? Is it possible that the person is daydreaming? Could they be looking at their phone? Is there a pedestrian who has not cleared the crossing? Why would someone who does not even know you want to mess up your day? Which is more likely, that the other driver is deliberately trying to upset you, or that they are simply not paying attention? By considering these other possible explanations, it becomes evident that the first thought is a thinking error. There is little or no evidence that the driver in front of you is deliberately trying to mess up your day.

Determining if the second thought noted is a thinking error is perhaps a bit more challenging. If you are at the end of a long line of vehicles and the light stays green for a relatively brief period, is it likely that you will miss the light? Alternatively, if you are close to the front of the line and the light tends to remain green for a relatively long period of time, then is it more likely you will still get through the light? In this case, more information is needed to determine whether you are engaged in a thinking error. However, in the absence of more information about the situation, the person described may not have much evidence that he will actually miss the light. If that is the case, then he is likely jumping to a conclusion.

The third thought is clearly a thinking error. If you have to wait until the next light, will it be the end of the world? Missing a green light and having to wait until the next one is an inconvenience, not a catastrophe.

In brief, the process of changing your thinking involves a three-step process:

1. Monitor by observing what you think and tell yourself.
2. Challenge and question what you think and tell yourself.
3. Replace thinking errors with alternative thoughts that are more accurate, realistic, in your best interests and that will reduce the risk of engaging in harmful behaviors.

You can also categorize your thoughts in terms of specific types of thinking errors. Categorizing thinking patterns allows you to more easily identify common types of thinking errors. These types of thinking errors regularly happen to many of us. Here are some common types of thinking errors.

1. **Overgeneralization** – Taking one event and applying it to all similar situations, assuming that they will all be the same. Taking a problem you have had with someone and thinking it applies to everyone else. Here are some examples:

    *   *Thinking **all** police are out to get you after you had a particularly bad experience with one police officer.*
    *   *Telling your partner that they **never** listen to you.*
    *   *Thinking your life will **never** get better after recent setbacks.*
    *   *Thoughts that include words like 'always' and 'never.'*

To replace overgeneralization, look for the exception. For example, you have had setbacks in the past, but things did improve over time.

2. **Black and White Thinking** – Thinking in absolutes. Judging someone or something as all good or all bad. Refusing to recognize the reality that nothing is 100% good or 100% bad. *You tend to think of things in extremes; either you are perfect or you're a total failure, right or wrong, win or lose.* Here are some examples:

    *   *Thinking that you are worthless because of a mistake you made.*

- *If I can't do something right, I should not bother to do it at all.*
- *You masturbated while trying to be abstinent, so you tell yourself that you should just give up because you are a failure.*

To replace black and white thinking look for the "gray" or look for the middle ground. For example, you may have made a mistake, but you have other qualities that make you a worthwhile person.

3. **Labeling** – This involves labeling someone or something with a word or a set of characteristics. You attach negative labels to yourself, others and the world. Here are some examples:

- *Thinking someone is jerk because they cut you off in traffic, ignoring the fact that that one act is only a part of who that person is.*
- *Look for thoughts that involve thinking of someone/something as a jerk, idiot, worthless or some similar pejorative label.*
- *Your friend cancels an appointment with you, and you think that he is lazy.*

To replace labeling, it is helpful to remember that people are more than just a label. We all have strengths and weaknesses that contribute to our overall character. This is particularly important as you are trying to change your sexual behaviors and improve your lifestyle. You are more than your past sexual choices.

4. **Jumping to Conclusions** – Taking a fact and making assumptions about what that fact means without getting further information. Here are some examples:

- *Thinking that someone is intending you harm because you didn't like what they said.*
- *Thinking someone does not like you because they have not called you back.*
- *Thinking someone is romantically interested in you because they smiled at you.*

To replace jumping to conclusions, think about other possible reasons for what has occurred. For example, is it possible that your friend did not call you back because they simply forgot or got busy?

5. **Catastrophizing** – Blowing a problem out of proportion, making it bigger than it really is. This thinking often leads to anxiety, and it can also lead to anger. Here are some examples:

- *Having lost my job is terrible; there is no hope now. This is the worst thing that could happen. My life is screwed.*
- *The government put wrong information in my file and there is no way to change it, so it is stuck with me forever and my life is ruined.*

To replace catastrophizing, ask yourself how bad is it? Is it really the end of the world, or simply a really tough and unpleasant situation? Can you see the problem in its relative scope within your life rather than as an all-encompassing problem?

6. **Musterbation/Shoulding** – This involves using words like "have to", "gotta", "must", "can't" and "should". Telling yourself that things have to go a certain way, that you must do something or that others must do something. A strong belief or expectation about how things "should" be. Look for this thinking pattern when your anger increases. This

thinking error leads to expectations and judgments about yourself and others. Here are some examples:

- *I have to do better than everyone else.*
- *They can't treat me this way.*
- *People shouldn't drive like that.*
- *They can't tell me what to do.*

To replace shoulding, change the "should" to a preference. For example, "I would *prefer* it if people drove slower/more quickly". In fact, when we look at the examples here, they are all preferences. It can be useful to remind yourself that you do not control other people or the world.

7. **Fear of Zero State** – Fear of being exposed as nothing, as unimportant to others. Many people who struggle with this thinking error believe "If I am not something, then I am nothing". Here are some examples:

   - *If I do not do well in this assignment, everyone will know I am really a loser.*
   - *I am a good person because of my relationship, and if I lose my relationship then I am worthless.*
   - *I have to show everyone how tough I am, or they will think I am a nothing.*

To replace fear of zero state thinking, consider what other things make you a worthy person. Look at your strengths. Consider the positive feedback that you have received from others.

8. **Positive mental filter** – Only seeing what you want to see in a certain situation, not seeing what is actually occurring. This thinking error leads people to avoid dealing with problems, ignoring problems or disregarding obvious things that require attention. Here are some examples of a positive mental filter:

   - *I have been unhappy in this relationship for a long time, but it's fine; it will work out in the end.*
   - *I can deal with this problem later.*
   - *Being told that you have strengths and weaknesses by your boss and only focusing on the strengths that you heard.*
   - *Ignoring a drug or alcohol problem by telling yourself, "It's fine, everyone drinks/uses drugs".*

It can be difficult to challenge positive mental filters because we use them to minimize or ignore problems. If you do not think that something is a problem, it is a good idea to ask a trusted friend for feedback about your perceptions. Ask yourself, is there something here I missed?

9. **Victim Stance** – Seeing yourself as a victim of the situation and not admitting your role in the situation. Believing because of what happened to you, you had no choice but to do what you did. It is important to not confuse victim stance with having actually been victimized. Here are some examples of victim stance thinking:

   - *It was their fault . . . they started it.*
   - *I don't deserve a speeding ticket – go find a real criminal.*

- *Why does this shit always happen to me?*
- *What happened to me isn't fair, so screw you!*

To challenge victim stance thinking, consider what role you played in the situation. Take responsibility for your part within the situation.

10. **Self-focused thinking** – Only seeing situations from your own point of view. Disregarding other people's perceptions of a situation. Thinking about yourself most of the time. Not considering how your actions might impact others. Here are some examples of self-focused thinking patterns:

- *What about my needs?*
- *I don't think that there is a problem, so there is not a problem.*
- *Rules don't apply to me.*

To challenge self-focused thinking, consider situations from other people's perspectives. What do others need in this situation? How would someone else perceive this situation? Try to put yourself in someone else's shoes.

11. **What-if thinking** – Being focused on what might happen rather than what is happening around you. This thinking pattern tends to enhance feelings of anxiety. Being focused on what might happen can be useful; for example, when we are looking at the potential consequences of using CSEM. However, if you overuse what-if thinking, you may find yourself worrying about all sorts of situations that may not happen to you. Here are some examples of what-if thinking:

- *I want to ask that girl out on a date, but what if she says no?*
- *I would apply for a job but what if they don't like me?*
- *What if I rebuild my life and someone finds out about my CSEM use? There is no point in trying.*

To counter what-if thinking, it will be important to look at the pros and cons of your decisions. Will this decision lead you to being happier and healthier in the future? We don't control what might happen tomorrow. We don't control how others react. Letting go of what-if thinking patterns involves ceasing to try to control the future. We can only make the best decisions for ourselves for today.

12. **Mindreading** – Telling yourself that you know how people think and feel without checking with them. This leads to problems when you begin to assume how people think and feel. Here are some examples of mindreading:

- *I know that she hates me.*
- *She always thinks that she is better than me.*
- *My boss thinks I am useless.*

Managing mindreading is very straightforward. You just need to get more information. Notice your assumptions and check with the other person. Ask questions. You may be surprised at what they tell you.

We all have thinking errors. These mistakes in our thinking happen all the time, and it is very common. The better you are at identifying, challenging and replacing yours, the more control you will have over your emotions and your behavior.

Behavioral Interventions

The behaviors we engage in can also help us to manage our emotions and urges. Indeed, when we become very upset, it can sometimes be particularly difficult to think about our thinking. Sometimes we need to slow our body down before we can focus on our thinking. We won't look at every behavioral intervention, but let's look at a few of the more commonly used strategies.

The focus when using behavioral interventions is to change what we are doing. We change our behaviors to impact how we are feeling and thinking. There are many ways to change our behaviors. Here are some examples:

1) **Deep breathing.** The use of deep breathing seems like a very simple technique, yet many people never pay much attention to how their breathing influences their emotional arousal. Breathing can be used to reduce emotional arousal and upset. If you begin to pay attention to your breathing, you may notice that your breathing becomes short and shallow when you are anxious or upset. That tends to worsen anxiety, and anxiety can make it harder to think about your thinking. You are encouraged to practice the use of deep breathing on occasions where you find yourself becoming markedly anxious or angry. A simple breathing technique involves placing one hand on your chest and the other on your belly. Take a deep slow breath in through your nose, allowing your diaphragm (your belly, not your chest) to inflate with a full intake of air. Slowly exhale. Continue to take 6 to 10 deep, slow breaths per minute. You can do this in the midst of anxiety, and it is also recommended that you practice doing this for 10 minutes each day. Regular use of deep breathing can also help reduce your heart rate and blood pressure.

2) **Time outs.** There are occasions where we are so aroused and upset that it can be useful to escape the situation – in a healthy way. By this, we don't mean taking a drink of alcohol or a drug. Rather, it can be useful to take a 10- or 15-minute "time out". Taking a time out means that you retreat for a short period of time to use calming strategies. If you are in a social situation, it will be important to let the other person know you are not running away but you simply need a few minutes to calm down before returning to deal with the situation. During your time out, it is important to use deep breathing and begin to examine your thinking and possible thinking errors.

3) **Exercise.** This intervention is not always practical in a high-stress situation, but it can very be useful to integrate into your daily life. Regular cardiovascular exercise helps to reduce anxiety, enhances mood and enhances your ability to think well. Exercise can make you more resilient in the face of day-to-day challenges. Practice exercising daily, ideally for at least 20–30 minutes. Get your heart rate up. This will help you better manage your thinking and emotions. Remember to check with your health care professional prior to starting a new exercise program.

4) **Talking to a trusted person.** In the midst of a difficult emotional experience, it can be useful to talk to someone you trust. It is important that you choose someone who is a positive support and who generally tends to improve your mood in the face of challenges. When we are physically close to people that we love and trust, there is a reduction in stress hormones in the body. Also, if you are confiding in a positive support, that person may help you identify problematic ways of thinking and thereby help you identify and challenge any possible thinking errors. Talking to someone can help!

5) **Mindfulness.** Practicing mindfulness can be a useful way to address your physical arousal levels and your mood. Mindfulness means being completely present in the moment and allowing yourself to feel your feelings, without judgment and without

trying to fix that feeling. There are many ways to practice mindfulness. Look for mindfulness apps, courses, groups and/or videos to assist you in learning mindfulness practice. We encourage you to integrate mindfulness practice in your daily life!

Behavioral interventions are very useful. While they appear to be simple, behavioral interventions can be hard to put in place consistently. They require regular practice. The more you practice these skills, the easier the skills will be to use when you really need them. Practicing behavioral interventions is important. If you don't use them, if you are not comfortable applying them or if you don't practice them, they won't work.

Sometimes it feels hard to do the things that you know will help you feel better. Often, we know that we need to exercise, care for ourselves, eat right, but in the moment, we don't make those helpful choices. Remember that change involves the consistent application of new skills. It doesn't have to be perfect, but every day that you try gets you closer to your goals. The more you do new things, helpful things, the more you are moving toward change.

Ensuring that you are exercising, talking to supports and calming your body down when you are upset are important skills. Identify some behavioral interventions that you think will be helpful for you and which you think you can reliably integrate into your life.

1. _____

_____

2. _____

_____

3. _____

_____

4. _____

_____

5. _____

_____

6. _____

_____

Pharmacological Interventions

There are situations where managing your thinking and behaviors can be augmented with medication to help with mood or impulses. It can be difficult to apply oneself to change if you are suffering from a mental health problem. There are medications that can help with mental health problems like anxiety and depression. There are also medications that can be useful if you are struggling with ADHD, drug or alcohol abuse. It is important to consult your physician regarding whether you are an appropriate candidate for medication that can help with your mental health.

If you are struggling with strong sexual urges and fantasy, there are medications that can help reduce sex drive and fantasy. Indeed, some of the medications that are used to treat depression actually help to reduce sex drive. There is also a class of medications referred to as anti-androgens that can assist you if other medication options haven't helped to reduce strong sexual urges and fantasy. Anti-androgens are typically used in situations where a "stronger" medication is seen as necessary. Of course, medications can have side effects and it is important to consider the benefits as well as potential costs of using medication. Speak with your physician about potential side effects and consider what is right for you.

Sometimes people believe that using medication should be avoided because they believe that they should be able to do it alone, without the help of medication. Mental health issues can be influenced by our biology, and there are occasions where medication can be an important part of treatment and a step toward a healthier life.

I plan to consult with my physician to discuss medications. Yes _____/No _____

When discussing medications with my physician, my goals are:

_____

_____

_____

_____

_____

Let's practice what you learned in this chapter. Use the following template to identify your thinking errors, create replacement thoughts that are more useful to you and practice some new behavioral interventions.

1) Notice your thinking errors and fill out the following grid.
2) Practice a new behavioral intervention.
3) Evaluate how this process worked for you. What was most helpful?
4) Do this daily to practice and maintain change.
5) Share your progress with your treatment provider.

Make as many copies of this sheet as you need, or use another notebook or journal to track your progress. Don't forget to congratulate yourself on your efforts for using these new skills!

Day _____ Date_____
Situation

_____

_____

_____

_____

Thoughts: Type of Thinking Error

1. _____

   _____

2. _____

_____

3. _____

_____

4. _____

_____

5. _____

_____

Replacement Thought (Each thinking error needs a rationale replacement)

1. _____

_____

2. _____

_____

3. _____

_____

4. _____

_____

5. _____

_____

Behavioral Interventions that I practiced today

1. _____

_____

2. _____

_____

3. _____

_____

4. _____

_____

5. _____

_____

Outcome: I felt:

_____

_____

_____

_____

_____

_____

In the next chapter, we will start examining your sexual management in more detail.

CHAPTER SUMMARY

- Managing your thinking involves monitoring your thinking, challenging your thinking errors and replacing your thinking errors through the use of more rationale replacement thoughts.
- It is important to be able to distinguish between a situation, a thought, an emotion and a behavior.
- Thinking errors can be categorized into various types. Knowing what type of thinking error you are engaged in can help with identifying an appropriate replacement thought.
- Behavioral interventions are another important part of change. It is used in conjunction with managing your thinking.
- Medication can also be an important part of treatment. Consult with your physician or a psychiatrist for additional assistance.

REFERENCES

Beck, A. (1963). Thinking and depression. I. Idiosyncratic content and cognitive distortions. *Archives of General Psychiatry*, *9*(4), 324–333.

5

Fantasy Management

CLINICIAN GUIDE

Throughout this chapter, we focus on talking openly and clearly about sexuality. In particular, we explore the sexual fantasies that relate to the client's use of child sexual exploitation material.

In your work with the client, start by discussing fantasy, sexual thoughts and sexual urges. Clearly defining the concepts of fantasy and sexual urges is very important. Frequently, clients will have a different understanding of the words fantasy, sexual fantasy and urges. Using the word *sexual thoughts* or *images/pictures/films in your mind* can be helpful alternatives. Start with creating an understanding of how your client defines sexual fantasy. Use their words to ensure that you understand their perception of these concepts. Then work on clarifying these concepts in ways that resonate with your client. Ensure that both you and the client understand the meaning and application of these concepts as it relates to communicating their sexual thoughts, feelings and behaviors.

As you explore the various types of sexual thoughts the client is experiencing, start introducing the concept of monitoring or journaling their sexual thoughts and urges. Invite the client to start identifying their sexual thoughts and assessing the frequency and intensity of these sexual thoughts. Such monitoring can help clients better understand the emotional and situational factors that can influence sexual thoughts and urges and the link to problematic behavior. The importance of tracking sexual urges with a log begins early in treatment and needs to be clearly explained. This information will allow you to tailor the treatment plan to the client and monitor treatment effectiveness. The knowledge of when your client is struggling the most, the context of these struggles and the resulting behaviors is essential for you to know. It will directly impact your treatment plan. The sexual log is essential to give you accurate information about your client's treatment needs. By identifying ongoing sexual thoughts and fantasy, you are actively addressing treatment effectiveness and you ensure that the client and their treatment efforts stay on track.

Clearly determine when the client is experiencing thoughts of illegal sexual activities and differentiate those from thoughts about legal sexual activities. Break down their sexual behaviors to include various activities that create sexual arousal for them. This may include: Internet surfing for sexual content, sexual fantasy/sexual thoughts only, masturbation and/or various forms of sexual activity. This will help the client identify patterns in their own behaviors. Discuss the proportion of illegal vs legal content in their sexual fantasies. Ensure that the client is able to identify sexually arousing consensual sexual thoughts. Encourage

DOI: 10.4324/9781003388142-6

them to move from illegal content to legal/healthy thoughts and fantasies. Clearly discuss the importance of changing their patterns of reinforcement as it pertains to sexual orgasm and pleasure. Patterns of reinforcement need to be understood by clients and therapists. The link between thought/fantasy and orgasm matters. While changing these patterns can be difficult, it will offer the client feelings of success, particularly if they are feeling hopeless in their ability to change their arousal patterns.

Once the client can clearly outline the frequency of sexual urges and fantasies, the content of the fantasies as well as their typical behavioral choices following these urges, it is time to help the client try various interventions to address their behaviors. At times, some clients get sidetracked by wanting to explore the "why" of their behaviors. They seek explanations for their choices, rather than focusing on behavioral change. We encourage you to monitor for this tendency and to redirect the client to work on direct behavioral change rather than taking an explanatory approach. At least initially, exploring the "why" does not lead to positive shifts in behaviors. Over time, your client will better understand their risk factors and, as they complete treatment modules, will better conceptualize their offending behaviors. Initially, creating behavioral change is most helpful to engaging clients and creating hope and pride in their treatment progress.

One intervention is to put Internet monitoring software on all their devices. This may also extend to their work devices. Monitoring software limits the ability for people to search online sexual content. Ideally, it also offers an accountability feature where all online searches are directly sent to a third party for accountability and review. Ask your client to identify an accountability partner, friend or family member who can serve as a witness to their online choices. Frame this positively to the client. It helps keep them safe by creating accountability and verification, which also builds trust within their community. Their positive choices are noted and encouraged. Also, if there is any question about their online choices, this can be clearly demonstrated and proven in an objective way. Finally, if they are facing a particularly strong urge, external barriers can help assist them to make a different choice in the moment.

There are many different types of monitoring software. Some are marketed to those wanting to cease pornography use, some are marketed to those wanting to reduce overall screen time and some are marketed to families. As long as the software blocker can provide both an external barrier (no sexualized content or no cellphone use after 10pm, for example) and accountability (tracking of your online activities to an accountability partner), then the program can be useful.

Here are a few examples:

- X3Watch
- Lion
- Truple
- NetNanny
- Accountable2You
- EverAccountable
- Pluckeye
- Qustodio
- MM Guardian
- Our Pact
- Boomerang

Note that there are other parental control software programs available. The list of available services tends to change frequently. Get to know these types of programs and find one that you are comfortable recommending to your clients.

In this portion of the treatment, ensure that you discuss concrete ways to manage sexual urges. Clients may have already discovered ways that work for them. Talk about alternative ways to manage their urges, including distractions, affirmations and reminders, talking to an accountability partner, remembering the consequences and introducing healthy sexual thoughts. There are many types of distractions. These can include exercise, new hobbies, additional work projects or goals, building their community involvement, volunteer work, music, food or other activities that distract them from the intensity of their urges.

Discussing the consequences of offending is another way to help clients consider a different point of view as it relates to their sexual choices. We will get into this in more detail in the following chapters, but for now, we will start to integrate the idea of consequences, either for themself, their loved ones or the victims as one way to make different choices. The inclusion of healthy sexual thoughts can also help the client make positive sexual choices. Healthy sexual thoughts include finding ways to promote legal sexual choices. One example would be to create consensual sexual scenarios that are arousing for the client as well as addressing sexual concerns which may be related to sexual performance or sexual orientation. Use their log to determine the intensity of various sexual thoughts and urges and to help find alternative thoughts that would also work well for them.

For some clients, creating a brief time to stop all sexual behaviors can help them reintroduce sexuality into their lives in a healthier way. This is particularly true of clients who struggle with sexual preoccupation or sex as a way of coping with stressors or emotions. The client's fantasy logs will inform you whether or not this is an appropriate strategy for your client. Each client is different. For example, you may not want to use this strategy with an overcontrolled client or with a client who is able to shift their masturbation habits and engage sexually with a consenting adult partner. We include this treatment option for you to explore with your client as it can be helpful for some CSEM clients. As with everything in this workbook, ensure that you tailor the treatment plan to meet each client's individual needs.

We will continue to discuss sexuality, sexual fantasy and sexual performance issues among other sexual topics in more detail in Chapter 8. Ensure that you discuss what is sexually exciting and arousing for the client, rather than dictating what sex "should" be. Keeping an open mind within this chapter and getting to know your client's sexual preferences will build better discussions about how to create a sex life that they can maintain moving forward. If your client is significantly struggling with managing their fantasies, it may be useful to explore undiagnosed mental health conditions, executive functioning deficits and/or other difficulties that enhance impulsivity and can lead to poor self-control. We encourage you to continue exploring these possibilities while also offering additional interventions to create some success in the treatment process.

An additional intervention to help your client achieve success with their fantasy management is olfactory reconditioning (Campbell-Fuller & Craig, 2009). Olfactory reconditioning is an intervention based on basic behavioral reinforcement principles. This approach has been discussed for many years in the professional literature (see Laws, 2001 for details). In short, when the client is having a sexual fantasy, they would use a noxious smell to interrupt their sexual arousal. The AversX company offers products and procedures to assist people with unwanted behaviors by applying these principles (see http://aversx.com for details). It has been our experience that, for some clients, simply having an alternative way to manage a sexual fantasy can have some clinical benefits. We encourage you to obtain clinical consultation and supervision prior to integrating these approaches in your practice.

Another option we encourage you to consider is to send the client for psychiatric consultation to discuss the use of sex drive-reducing medications when they are struggling with managing their sexual thoughts and fantasies. Medications can be helpful to reduce the frequency and intensity of sexual fantasy. This can be a helpful option for clients who struggle with ongoing sexual preoccupation. As always, working productively with your client to explore their intervention options is an important part of the treatment plan.

Be curious when working with the client on the materials presented in this chapter. There are many ways to establish a healthy and interesting sex life. Discuss these in detail, and if you are uncertain about the direction that the client is taking in regard to their sexual choices, refer to your colleagues and professional consultation group for feedback and suggestions.

REFERENCES

Campbell-Fuller, N., & Craig, L. (2009). The use of olfactory aversion and directed masturbation in modifying deviant sexual interest: A case study. *Journal of Sexual Aggression*, *15*(2), 179–191. https://doi.org/10.1080/13552600902759556

Laws, D. R. (2001). Olfactory aversion: Notes on procedure, with speculations on it's mechanism of effect. *Sexual Abuse: A Journal of Research and Treatment*, *13*(4), 275–287.

CLIENT WORKBOOK

Learning Objectives

In this chapter, you will:

a) Learn the definition of the word *fantasy*
b) Identify why understanding fantasies is important to managing CSEM use
c) Identify the benefits of using a fantasy log
d) Understand the importance of using Internet monitoring software to avoid sexual content online
e) Understand the importance of healthy sexual fantasies
f) Address stubborn sexual fantasies that won't go away

In this chapter, we want to help you understand the link between sexual fantasy and the use of unhealthy sexual behaviors, including accessing CSEM.

Let's start by defining what we mean. What is a fantasy? Fantasies are pictures in your head, words in your head or thoughts in your head that are sexual or non-sexual in nature and may reflect your interest in illegal sexual activities. These pictures or thoughts can be easy to notice, like watching a full-length movie, or they can be difficult to notice, like a passing thought that quickly zips through your mind. Fantasizing is an act of the imagination that may be represented in images or thoughts. The content, duration and intensity of a fantasy can vary. Fantasies can involve memories of past events or purely imagined scenarios that are outside your direct experience. In fact, many people fantasize about things they have not done. A fantasy can be deliberately brought to mind, or it may simply appear. The nature of the fantasy may be welcome, or it can cause distress. In this workbook, we are focusing on fantasies that serve to perpetuate your sexual interests and sexual thoughts.

> A sexual fantasy is any thought or image that is sexual in nature. Looking at something or someone that arouses you, running a sexual scenario in your head, thinking about sex and identifying a potential sexual partner are all examples of sexual fantasy.

Fantasies can have a profound effect on how we feel, the urges that we have, and what we do! Addressing your fantasy life is very important. Often, people do not realize how much fantasy runs their lives. Fantasy can be one of the early warning signs before problematic behavior occurs. This chapter is about helping you monitor and manage your fantasies. As you begin to monitor your fantasies, it will be helpful to think of them in regard to:

• The content: What are you thinking about?
• The frequency: How often do you have this fantasy?
• The duration: How long does the fantasy last?
• The intensity: How real does the fantasy feel?

Think about your favorite meal. What does it include? How does it taste? How does it feel in your mouth? How do you feel when you are eating it?

As you were beginning to imagine your favorite meal, what did you notice? Did you salivate a bit? Did you have the taste in your mouth? Did you have an urge to go and get it from the fridge?

Say you do this on a regular basis. What will happen?

Without quite knowing how you got there, you will be sitting in front of your favorite meal. You have tightened the link between a positive experience and that particular food. Fantasy works in a similar fashion.

Notice where you are allowing your mind to go, then create a new path for your thoughts!

It is important to understand that when you masturbate to a fantasy, you make the fantasy more intense. There is a link between behavior and fantasy. It is important to identify and address this link. It is normal for people to fantasize. It becomes a concern when fantasy interferes with healthy functioning, contributes to poor choices and leads to engaging in unhealthy and illegal behaviors, including the viewing of CSEM. As we begin to talk about your use of fantasy, it is important to consider the content of your fantasies.

You may be thinking: "Isn't it normal for people to think about sexual things?" or "Aren't people thinking about sex 24/7?" or "How can a fantasy be a problem? It is just a thought in my head".

Healthy sexual fantasies follow the rules of sexual consent. They involve adults. There is no difference in power between the participants, and everyone is sober, awake and conscious. All participants are able to consent and have consented to the sexual activities.

Healthy sexual fantasies are not about you when you were a child or a teenager. Even if the person in the fantasy is a younger version of you, it is still unhealthy because you are a child in your own mind.

Healthy sexual fantasies are consensual and age-appropriate. What you think about matters. What you think about when you have a positive sexual experience, like an orgasm, matters a lot!

At times, people get lost asking, "Why? Why do I have these thoughts? Why is this happening to me?" Asking *why* can keep you stuck. It often leads to getting lost in the past. While it can be tempting to become focused on why you have these fantasies, it may not be helpful to you as a first step in managing this problem. When working on this issue, your first step is not to focus on *why*. The focus is on *what* and *when*.

Here are more helpful questions to ask yourself when you are trying to change:

"What are my fantasies about?"
"When do they become more frequent?"
"When do they become more intense?"
"What are these fantasies doing to me?"
"When do they last longer?"
"What practical tools will I use to change this pattern?"

Your first task is to notice what is going on. Fantasy logs are a great tool for this. Every time you have a sexual thought, write it down in the log. There are many different ways to structure a fantasy log. _There is no right or wrong way – the goal is to find an approach that works for you_. In the next pages, you will see three different versions of a sexual fantasy log. Use the fantasy log structure that works for you, or create your own.

A good sexual fantasy log includes: the date, time of day, context for the event, nature of the sexual thought (was it legal or illegal?), action (whether you masturbated or not), your feelings at that time and the intensity of the fantasy (you can identify intensity on a rating scale from 1 to 10: 1 is a passing fantasy, 5 a moderately engaging fantasy and 10 is an extremely intense fantasy). If you need privacy, you can design your log so that your private information is not obvious to others who may inadvertently see your log (see example #3 for details).

It is important to understand that when you masturbate to a fantasy, you reinforce it; you make that fantasy more intense. This is why the fantasy log is so important. You need to notice your sexual fantasies and thoughts about children and change them; you need to stop masturbating to thoughts of children. We will talk more about this later in this chapter.

Fantasy log – Template #1: Table

Fill out each column of information

Date	Time of day	Context	L or I (Legal or Illegal)	M (Masturbated?) Yes or No	Intensity 1–10	Feelings

Fantasy Log – Template #2: Journal Entry

Information should include:

Date; time of day; context (what is going on right now?); nature of the fantasy (legal or illegal? *Do not provide excessive details, as it is important not to make journaling an arousing activity*). Describe the intensity of the fantasy. Did you masturbate? How much time did you spend engaging in the fantasy/masturbation? How were you feeling before the fantasy/masturbation? How were you feeling afterward? Make note of any other information that you think is important, such as substance use or mental health symptoms.

When journaling, it is important to review your journal entries regularly to look for patterns. Try to do this every few days. Simply journaling without exploring your journal for patterns will likely not be as helpful to you.

Example:

Date: Thursday August 31

I woke up this morning feeling unmotivated to go to work. I stayed in bed under the covers. I had an erection and started thinking about sex. I thought about porn images I had seen about female adults and kids. I started to masturbate, but then decided to stop. The intensity of the fantasy was moderate. It was possible to stop, get up, and go have breakfast instead. Before the fantasy, I felt sad. After I got up and had breakfast, I felt more motivated to start my day.

Date: Friday September 1

I had a crazy busy day at work. My boss was a total ass. I came home and felt angry. I had a sexual thought about porn images I had seen involving children. I masturbated. The intensity of the fantasy was pretty strong. I was feeling angry before I masturbated. I felt better right after I was done, but then I felt so awful. I felt guilty and shitty.

Fantasy Log – Template #3: Coded Journal Entry

If you are concerned about somebody reading your journal, make your own code to represent each section. Write whatever works for you, as long as you keep track of what each symbol means. Check each box that corresponds to your code.

In this example, the code is: Legal = Y; Illegal = N; Intensity = 1 to 10 (1 passing fantasy, 5 moderately engaging fantasy, 10 extremely intense fantasy); Masturbation? = M; Positive feelings = +; Negative feelings = –, Time of day = am or pm.

Date:
Y
N
1–10
M
+
–
am
pm

Example using the context from journal log template #2:

Date: *Thursday August 31*
Y ✓
N ✓
1–10 5
M ✓
+
– ✓
am ✓
pm
Date: *Friday September 1*
Y
N ✓
1–10 8
M ✓
+
– ✓
am
pm ✓

Use a fantasy log to monitor your behavior and identify patterns. As you begin monitoring your fantasies, you may notice that you use masturbation to get yourself going in the morning, or perhaps you use masturbation to slow yourself down at the end of the day. Sometimes people use masturbation to deal with feelings of boredom or loneliness. Others use it as a reward when good things happen in their lives. You may notice that you prefer using CSEM to create and maintain sexual arousal. As you increase your awareness, what patterns emerge?

These are the patterns that I notice in my fantasy log:

_____

_____

_____

_____

_____

Allowing thoughts of illegal sexual behaviors to happen can lead to trouble! What you tell yourself when you have such thoughts is a topic that we will tackle in a later chapter. If you are reading this workbook, it is likely that you have already had thoughts of illegal sexual behaviors. These sexual thoughts may have been very comforting for a long time, seeming like a safe place to retreat. You can understand these as being either thoughts or fantasies. The notion of giving these thoughts up may result in some mixed feelings for you. You may want to change your thoughts, but there may also be a part of you that wants to keep them. As you struggle with this, it may be helpful to ask yourself whether these thoughts have really made your life better. Have they really made life healthier for you? Have they moved you toward the life that you want to have? It will be important to face these questions to move from simply monitoring your thoughts and fantasies to putting the effort into managing and changing these thoughts and fantasies. You may also want to re-examine the questions in Chapter 2 again to fully explore your motivation for change. See the following exercise to explore this theme in more detail.

Exercise: The impact of sexual thoughts about children

What impact have sexual fantasies about children and underage youths had on my life?
Short term: _____

_____

_____

Long term: _____

_____

_____

What impact have sexual fantasies about children and underage youths had on how I feel about myself?
Short term: _____

_____

_____

Long term: _____

_____

_____

How have sexual fantasies about children and underage youths helped me manage my emotions?

Short term: _____

_____

_____

Long term: _____

_____

_____

What impact have sexual fantasies about children and underage youths had on my relationships with others?

Short term: _____

_____

_____

Long term: _____

_____

_____

What would life look like if I was not engaging in these types of fantasies?

Short term: _____

_____

_____

Long term: _____

_____

_____

The more you know about when and how often you fantasize, the easier it will be to change. We will start with noticing when fantasies happen and how often. When it happens, write it down. Don't give up! Tracking your behavior is the first step to understanding your patterns and <u>changing</u> your patterns. You want to change, so don't be afraid to write it down! If you are not in a private place where you can safeguard your writings, use fantasy log template # 3 (see earlier example) and create a code that you understand to help you monitor your behaviors.

> *When you are using your fantasy log, it is important not to go into great detail outlining your sexual fantasies. You don't want to make the content sexually arousing! Your log is a way to hold yourself accountable. For example, "Yes, I had this thought today. Yes, I masturbated today". Make sure that you don't allow yourself to make completing the fantasy log sexually stimulating.*

Now let's talk about the patterns that emerge in your fantasy log. Everyone is different. Acknowledging these patterns begins the process of identifying the contexts that are related to your use of sexual fantasy. This is very important. Many people use sexual fantasy, sexual activity and orgasm as a way to feel better. This may be you, too.

Fred finds himself thinking about sex often, independent of the context that he is in during the day (at work, at home, at the mall). He thinks about sex when he is angry, happy and sad. His sexual thoughts range from sexual activities with adults all the way to having sex with children.

Joe notices that he has sexual fantasies when he is stressed and upset. It tends to get worse when he feels rejected.

Mike engages in sexual fantasies that almost always involve sexual thoughts about children.

As you notice your patterns, you may notice that certain emotions trigger your fantasies (for example, loneliness, anxiety, sadness or even happiness), that some beliefs trigger your fantasies (e.g., "This will help me feel better" or "Nobody is getting hurt") or that sexual excitement (e.g., experiencing intense sexual urges) contributes to your fantasies. If you find that emotions trigger your fantasies, how can you begin to manage these emotions in other ways? If you notice that relationship problems trigger fantasies for you, what can you do to develop satisfying relationships? If you notice that you often have sexual thoughts about children or about past sexual images of children that you have viewed online, what can you do to change your sexual thoughts? If you notice that your sexual excitement propels you forward, how can you interrupt this process? What if you notice that watching any sort of pornography triggers you to move from sexual thoughts about adults to children? Discuss your observations with your treatment provider.

If your pattern is not clear, track it for a longer period of time. If it still isn't clear, talk to your treatment provider and review your logs together.

Hopefully, you have identified the benefits of managing problematic sexual fantasies. Here are several ways to gain control over sexual fantasies rather than allowing sexual fantasies to have control over you. Let's fight those inappropriate thoughts!

Deciding To Stop Focusing on Sexual Thoughts. STOP!

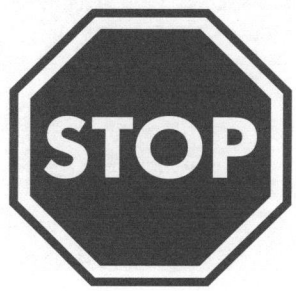

If you have noticed that sexuality has become a very large part of your life, start with abstinence. Cease all masturbation and sexual thoughts. It is time for a break. This is a break, not a sexual ban for life. For right now, no masturbation, no fantasy. Get out of situations where you might have taken the time to fantasize and masturbate in the past. This may involve restructuring your daily routine so that you do not have the time or space to indulge in fantasy and masturbation. The goal is for you to have a better understanding of how fantasy and masturbation play a role in your life and to reset your sexuality.

> Charles noticed that he masturbated in the morning. He was not regularly plagued with sexual fantasies at work, but he certainly struggled with these at the beginning of most days. He joined a morning jogging group so that he had to wake up and jump out of bed in the morning. He filled that time with a more productive activity. To his surprise, the urges that he usually experienced passed relatively quickly when he focused on exercise. He also enjoyed the jogging community and the new people that he met in his neighborhood.

External barriers can be very helpful in achieving your goal of abstinence from sexual fantasy and masturbation. *Internet monitoring software is available and can be used on all your electronic devices.* This software will limit your ability to access violent and sexual content. Various parental control software is available. Importantly, this type of software can send accountability reports to your assigned accountability partner. It will track where you go online and send those links to any person you choose. This way, you have a direct line of accountability. Accountability regarding your choices and behaviors is very important. We will talk more about accountability in Chapter 12.

Many people find community support programs very helpful in their goal of abstinence. Attending local programs such as SA (Sexaholics Anonymous), SAA (Sex Addicts Anonymous) or using online resources like Stop it NOW!, Don't Offend, No Fap and Virtuous Pedophiles can be good ways to find support in your efforts to change.

Remember: the goal is not long-term abstinence. The goal is to regain control over your sexuality and your sexual choices. Once you have more control, reintroducing healthy sexuality is the goal.

If I Have a Sexual Thought About a Child: Manage!

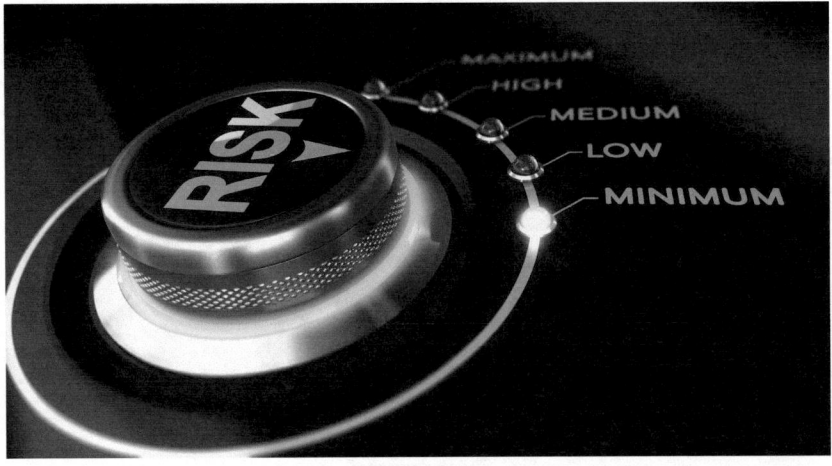

Manage your risk

If you do have a sexual thought about a child, the best approach is to stop it in its tracks. Drop your penis! Go do something else. Call a friend. Exercise. Get involved in another activity. Distraction can be very helpful in managing a sexual urge.

Examples of distractions:

What distractions would work best for you when you are facing an urge to fantasize or masturbate to a thought about a child? Write down your ideas.

_____

_____

_____

_____

Practice using these distractions this week.
Upon reflection, which ones worked the best?

_____

_____

_____

Continue to use the distractions that worked the best for you!

If Distraction Doesn't Work: Visualize the Consequences!

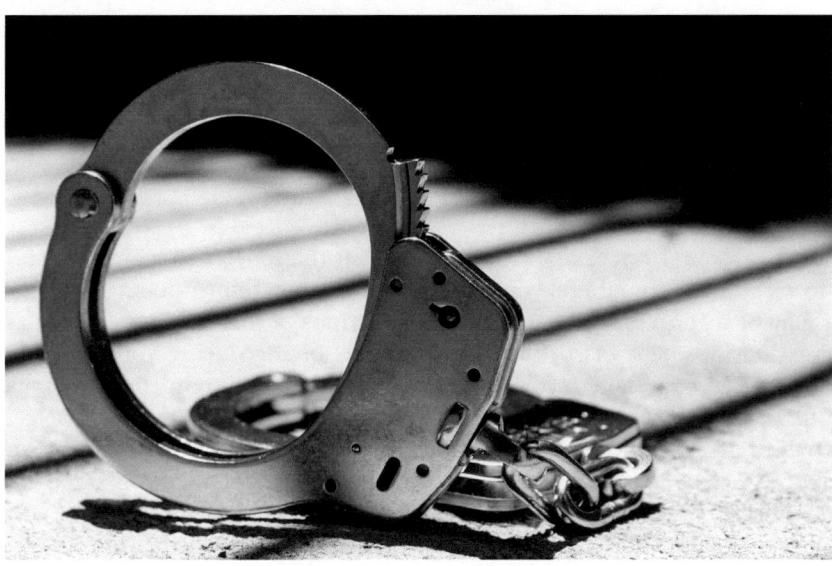

Remember the Consequences
When distraction is not enough, visualize the negative consequences that may happen to you if you continue down this road. Imagine your partner or your close friend discovering your online activities. Image them ending their relationship with you. Imagine yourself facing police at your door. Imagine the cold, hard feel of handcuffs. Imagine the reactions of your

loved ones, friends and family members to your arrest. Imagine the shame that you would feel if your name and picture were published in the media. Use these negative consequences to remember why you are working at changing your behaviors.

Describe in detail the possible legal consequences if you continue your fantasy. What will happen to you? Is it worth it?

_____

_____

_____

_____

_____

Another helpful strategy is to visualize the positive consequences of how you would feel if you do not use illegal sexual material. Imagine the pride and happiness that you would feel about your accomplishment. Use these positive consequences to remember why you are working at changing your behaviors.

Describe in detail the positive feelings that you would have if you didn't engage in your fantasy. How would you feel about yourself?

_____

_____

_____

_____

_____

_____

If you choose to abstain from sexual fantasy and masturbation, try to maintain this goal for at least four to six weeks. From there, you can determine when reintroducing sex will work best for you. It may be a good idea to work on other sections of this workbook, such as thinking patterns, relationships, sleep issues and/or problem-solving during your period of abstinence. When you feel ready, talk to your treatment provider about reintroducing masturbation into your life.

Masturbation is not bad. It can be a fun activity, either alone or with a partner. Creating and developing healthy, legal fantasies for yourself is essential. If you often have sexual thoughts involving children or other inappropriate sexual behavior, it will be important to create healthy sexual fantasies involving adults to use during masturbation.

Describe in detail a legal, consensual sexual adult fantasy that arouses you, meaning it turns you on. Use this fantasy to masturbate moving forward.

_____

_____

_____

_____

_____

Albert is using a legal consensual adult fantasy that he created to kick out those thoughts of illegal sexual behaviors about children. When he starts to masturbate to legal thoughts, he notices that his mind drifts and adds sexual thoughts about children to his adult scenario. What should he do?

It can be quite common to have difficulty keeping your sexual thoughts focused on adults, particularly if you have a long history of having sexual thoughts involving children. It is very important that you stop masturbating as soon as your fantasy is no longer legal or if it contains any non-consensual activities. If this is happening to you, focus on abstinence to enhance your practice of controlling your sexual thoughts and sexual behaviors before integrating healthy sexuality back into your life.

What is my plan if and when thoughts of illegal sexual behaviors creep into my healthy sexual fantasies? What will I do? Be specific.

_____

_____

_____

_____

_____

Don't masturbate to thoughts of illegal sexual behaviors. If they creep up, stop. Continue to read this workbook and develop your ability to manage your thoughts and fantasies so you can reach your goals.

Nourish Healthy Sexual Fantasies

We often talk about nourishing ourselves with food, education, friendships; this also applies to our sexuality. We can feed our sexuality with healthy or unhealthy things. As you reduce your use of thoughts involving children, you must replace those thoughts with positive alternatives. The goal is for you to create a happy, satisfying sex life for yourself. This includes creating healthy, legal and appropriate sexual fantasies. The fantasies that you have should encourage you to make good choices. Feeding thoughts about illegal sexual behaviors is a huge problem. Feeding these thoughts is a springboard to accessing child sexual exploitation material (CSEM). What would be a better alternative?

Jose spent too much time online watching pornography. He watched all types of pornography every day. When he was at work, he spent time thinking about the porn that he had watched the previous day. He began to think about sexual activities that involved children. These thoughts became more and more prominent when he thought about sex. Jose took a break from porn. He also created sexual fantasies about adults that he found very arousing, and he enjoyed using these to masturbate. Using legal fantasies became fun again.

As noted earlier in this chapter, healthy sexual fantasies follow the rules of sexual consent. They involve adults. There is no difference in power between the participants and everyone is sober, awake and conscious. All participants are able to consent, and have consented, to the sexual activities. Healthy sexual fantasies follow and respect the law.

Healthy sexual fantasies are not about you when you were a child or a teenager. Even if the person in the fantasy is a younger version of you, it is still unhealthy because you are a child in your own mind. In a healthy sexual fantasy, all participants are of legal age and able to consent to the sexual activity.

You may want to consider strategies like reminders, positive healthy images or stories that can encourage you to nourish yourself with positive sexuality.

What will help you continue to use healthy sexual fantasies?

1) _____

2) _____

3) _____

4) _____

5) _____

6) _____

You may find that a specific feeling is linked to using sexualized thoughts of children. How you manage your feelings can be related to your use of these thoughts. If this is the case, please refer to Chapter 6 to address your emotions management in more detail.

It can become a habit to give yourself permission to indulge in sexualized fantasies about children. If you notice that you have a habit of giving yourself permission to think about illegal sexual behaviors, please refer to Chapter 7.

If My Sexual Thoughts and Fantasies of Children Are Still Not Going Away: Enhanced Management!

Sometimes distraction is not enough. If you are struggling to manage sexual thoughts of children and stop these thoughts in their tracks, don't give up! Remind yourself that you spent many hours masturbating and ejaculating to sexual thoughts about children, and the positive link you have created between sexual thoughts and orgasm can make it tougher to stop.

One option is using a strong smell or a bad taste to help deter you. If you have ever struggled with nail biting, you may know that using a bitter nail polish will make your nails taste bad. If you use bitter nail polish consistently, you will likely stop biting your nails eventually. Using a bad smell to stop a sexual thought about a child works the same way. There are companies, such as AversX, that sell products that taste or smell bad to help you manage your fantasies. If you are struggling with a sexual fantasy that is not going away, if you feel an urge to masturbate to a fantasy of a child or if you still feel aroused by such a fantasy, take a small sniff of a bad odor. Your sexual arousal will likely cease in that moment. This can help you regain control. If you do not suffer from any nasal concerns, ammonia salts can have a similar impact. We do not recommend eating any bad-tasting items, with the exception of products specifically made and marketed for this purpose (for example, AversX oral products). This strategy can be challenging to implement, and we strongly recommend that you obtain the help of your treatment provider or a qualified professional before you try it.

Medication is another way to address ongoing sexual thoughts about children Exploring the use of anti-depressant medications (SSRIs) can be helpful to address resistant sexual fantasies. In addition, there is also a class of medications that can be used to effectively decrease your sexual urges. These medications are called anti-androgen medications. Talk to your physician or treatment provider for additional information about these treatment options.

It is important to note that obsessive thinking patterns and mental health difficulties can make it difficult to apply the management strategies listed here (see Chapter 3 for details). Pursue additional psychological or medical attention if your thoughts are not going away or are not being reduced to a manageable level.

During this chapter, if you were struggling with thoughts about past events in your life or childhood abuse, it may be time to talk to your treatment provider, a trusted clinical counselor or mental health professional for additional assistance. We will tackle these themes in Chapter 10.

We will continue to explore sexuality by reviewing the link between emotions and sex in the next chapter.

CHAPTER SUMMARY

- Sexual fantasy is any thought that is sexual in nature.
- Healthy sexual fantasies are legal and do not cause harm to yourself or others. Maintain only healthy sexual fantasies.
- What you allow yourself to fantasize about matters. Keep your sexual thoughts and fantasies legal.
- You may need to abstain from sexuality for a period of time to give yourself a chance to improve your sexual habits.
- Maintain a sexual fantasy log.
- Use Internet monitoring software to avoid sexual content online.
- Reach out to community and online support programs for additional assistance.
- Visualize the consequences of your continued CSEM use if you are struggling to manage your sexual thoughts about children.
- Talk to your treatment provider about the use of foul odors or medications to manage your thoughts and fantasies.

6

Dealing With Emotions and Sex

CLINICIAN GUIDE

Emotions management is an important treatment target. Clients who struggle with managing their emotions may have difficulty changing entrenched behaviors. Cognitive behavioral therapy (CBT) is an essential tool in helping clients to enhance their emotions management skills and to facilitate change. For clients who particularly struggle with emotions management, this chapter can be moved to the beginning of your treatment plan.

This chapter is designed to help clients increase their ability to identify their emotions and experience those emotions without engaging in negative behaviors. When people try to avoid certain emotions or ignore them, it can become harder to manage them in helpful ways. We encourage you to start by teaching the importance of identifying emotional states. This chapter includes an emotions list to help the client familiarize themselves with various emotions and to increase their emotional vocabulary. Reviewing these emotions can also occur by utilizing a simplified emotions list or a feelings wheel. There are many different emotions lists and feelings wheels available (see Willcox, 1982 for one example). A typical emotions list or a feelings wheel will describe varied emotional states and the connections between the different types of emotions. This is one technique that can be used to help the client identify their different emotional states. Encourage clients to explore their understanding of emotions by asking them to describe varied emotional experiences in their lives. An emotions log complements the sexual fantasy log and offers additional monitoring of the client's daily experiences. The emotions log will help you understand where to focus your interventions with the client as it relates to their ongoing emotions management needs.

Once clients can identify their emotions, the goal is to help them see the connections between their emotional states and their sexual thoughts, fantasies and behaviors. These patterns were likely highlighted in the last chapter as they related to their fantasy log. Focusing on these patterns can help clients see relationships and direct links between their emotional states and their sexual choices. In our clinical experience, this relationship, when highlighted and understood by clients, can accelerate the change process.

When discussing emotional regulation, ensure that you address how the client responds to both <u>positive</u> and <u>negative</u> emotional states. Remember that for some clients, happiness or celebratory states can also impact sexual choices and the intensity of their sexual urges. As such, exploring both positive and negative emotional states will be essential.

You may find that certain emotions have a more direct relationship to sexual activity for your client. For example, the emotions of sadness and loneliness can often be related to

DOI: 10.4324/9781003388142-7

sexual fantasies and urges. The concept of "sad + lonely + horny" is another way to introduce the concept of sex as coping. In our clinical opinion, these three emotional states tend to precede higher urge intensity. Take the time to explore these links and work directly with the emotions that seem to create the most direct relationship with the client's sexual choices.

It is important to help clients build their tolerance for difficult emotions. CBT approaches to emotions management are presented in this chapter and include behavioral strategies (deep breathing, exercise) as well as cognitive strategies (visualizations and challenging unhelpful thoughts). Exploring alternative approaches such as DBT skills, which are designed to help clients address uncomfortable emotional states (Linehan, 2015), as well as Acceptance and Commitment Therapy (Hayes, Strosahl, & Wilson, 1999, 2011), may also be helpful. In addition, concepts such as windows of tolerance (Siegel, 1999), somatic experiencing (Levine, 2010) and/or encouraging general mindfulness practice are additional ways to assist people to tolerate intense emotions. You may also wish to refer your client for additional mental health services if usual CBT principles are not leading to significant improvement. Be mindful that past trauma can impact treatment responsiveness. We are not advocating the start of trauma-specific therapy at this point in the treatment process; however, this subject will be explored in later chapters.

A quick word about anger: anger management can often be an important treatment target. You may encounter clients who tend to avoid anger or who engage in passive-aggressive expressions of anger. Addressing anger management with CBT skills is encouraged as part of your treatment plan. While it is beyond the scope of this workbook to address anger management interventions in significant detail, we encourage you to work productively with clients who present with specific difficulties related to anger management. Local anger management programs may also be of assistance, and we have provided specific resources to address anger management in the references section of this workbook.

Emotions matter! Taking the time to address the client's emotions, emotional expression and emotional management is an important addition to their treatment plan. Effective problem-solving often derives from the insights obtained in this chapter. Effective problem-solving will be discussed in more detail in Chapter 10.

REFERENCES

Hayes, S. C., Strosahl, K. D., & Wilson, K. G. (1999). *Acceptance and commitment therapy: An experiential approach to behaviour change*. New York, NY: Guilford Press.

Hayes, S. C., Strosahl, K. D., & Wilson, K. G. (2011). *Acceptance and commitment therapy: The process and practice of mindful change* (2nd ed.). New York, NY: Guilford Press.

Levine, P. A. (2010). *In an unspoken voice: How the body releases trauma and restores goodness*. Berkeley, CA: North Atlantic Books.

Linehan, M. M. (2015). *DBT skills training manual* (2nd ed.). New York: The Guilford Press.

Siegel, D. (1999). *The developing mind: Towards a neurobiology of interpersonal experience*. New York, NY: Guilford.

Willcox, G. (1982). The feeling wheel: A tool for expanding awareness of emotions and increasing spontaneity and intimacy. *Transactional Analysis Journal, 12*(4), 274–276. https://doi.org/10.1177/036215378201200411

CLIENT WORKBOOK

Learning Objectives

In this chapter, you will:

a) learn to identify your emotions
b) learn the difference between emotions and thoughts
c) learn the benefits of using an emotions log
d) develop an understanding of the relationship between your emotions and your sexuality
e) apply tools to deal with your negative emotions

Would you believe that managing emotions matters when managing sexual problems? Emotions are important to our sexual health. Let's talk more about the relationship between emotions and sex!

It may be obvious, but SEX FEELS GOOD! Really good. Seems like a no-brainer, right? The fact that sex feels good keeps us motivated to have it again and again. This is important for the survival of our species; however, it also has some downsides. When we are feeling bad, we want to feel better. Sometimes trying to feel better by identifying and dealing with our emotions, resolving problems, fixing relationships and communicating openly with the important people in our lives can seem overwhelming. A nice orgasm can deal with all those negative feelings easily without putting in all that work. So what's the problem? Just masturbate and feel better. It is an easy shortcut, but a short-term fix can create a long-term problem. By doing this, you do not address the initial problem. With time, you may notice that you stop making good sexual decisions because *you just need to feel better in that one moment*. This can be the start of problem behaviors.

> Curtis is a very social guy. He used to work in forestry camps, surrounded by lots of friends and acquaintances. Curtis lost his job. He didn't just lose his income, but he also lost his friends and his daily routine. He had no goals. This made him feel mad and sad. Unfortunately, Curtis didn't talk about that. He spent his days watching television, masturbating, and viewing more and more pornography. Over time, his use of pornography included various types of images, including sexual images of children.

It is not unusual for people who access CSEM to talk about being depressed as a reason for using this material. Some users who access CSEM identify doing so when they are feeling sad, down, hopeless, unmotivated, suicidal or angry. This scenario might seem familiar to you. Noticing your mood is important. When was the last time you felt happy? When did you last sing or hum to yourself? When did you last feel connected to your community? When was the last time you liked your life?

The last time that I felt truly happy with my life was:

_____

_____

_____

_____

_____

As you think about the last time you felt truly happy with your life, can you recall if your sexual behavior was different in any way from periods in your life when you have been unhappy, angry or without a sense of purpose in life? If so, then it becomes all the more important to have a good understanding of your emotions. Being able to identify your emotions and put a name to them is part of understanding your emotions.

Here is a list of some common emotions.

Positive emotions: Absorbed • Acceptance • Adoration • Admiration • Affection • Alert • Amazed • Amused • Anticipation • Appreciative • Awe • Bubbly • Buoyant • Calm • Carefree • Caring • Comfortable • Compassionate • Confident • Contemplative • Determined • Eager • Ecstatic • Excitement • Feisty • Fondness Happy • Hopeful • Inspired • Jolly • Joy • Motivated • Optimistic • Peaceful • Powerful • Proud • Reassured • Relaxed • Relief • Satisfaction • Strong • Thankful • Triumph • Trust • Upbeat • Zippy

Neutral emotions: Astonishment • Cautious • Complacent • Content • Mellow • Surprised

Negative emotions: Adrift • Afraid • Agitated • Aggravated • Anger • Annoyed • Antagonistic • Alone • Antsy • Anxious • Apprehensive • Ashamed • Awkward • Baffled • Bashful • Betrayed • Bewildered • Bitter • Boredom • Bothered • Brooding • Concerned • Confusion • Contempt • Cranky • Defeated • Depressed • Despair • Devastated • Disappointed • Disdain • Disgust • Disturbed • Edgy • Embarrassment • Envy • Excluded • Exhausted • Fear • Frightened • Frustrated • Furious • Grief • Hatred • Helpless • Hurt • Inadequate • Insecure • Intimidated • Irritated • Jealous • Lethargic • Lonely • Lost • Melancholic • Miserable • Mortified • Nervous • Numb • Outraged • Overwhelmed • Pathetic • Pessimistic • Powerless • Preoccupied • Rage • Rattled • Regret • Remorse • Resentment • Sadness • Scared • Shame • Spiteful • Stressed • Terrified • Trapped • Uncomfortable • Upset • Worry • Weak • Worthless

Notice how you feel about yourself in this moment. How do you feel right now?

Today, I feel: _____

_____

What is the difference between emotions and thoughts? Most emotions can be described in a single word (e.g., angry, sad). Emotions are typically felt in your body, whereas thoughts typically occur in your head, as a string of words. Let's see how this applies. If someone says, "I feel like he doesn't like me", is that a thought or a feeling? It is a thought because it is a string of words, not a bodily sensation. If my hands are clenched, my face is red and I am breathing fast, is this a thought or a feeling? These are reactions that indicate a feeling, likely anger. Continue to become more aware of your emotions as a first step to better managing your emotions and yourself.

We have indicators that help us identify our emotions. These indicators can be physical, behavioral or interpersonal.

Physical cues: Changes in your body that occur when you are feeling a particular emotion. For example, when you are anxious you may notice your face feeling hot, you might notice that you are shaking, your stomach is clenching or you might notice your teeth grinding.

Behavioral cues: Changes in your behaviors that occur when you are feeling a particular emotion. For example, you notice that your fists are clenched when you are angry, or you might notice yourself singing when you are happy.

Interpersonal cues: Changes in how you behave toward others. For example, if you are angry you might notice yourself saying mean or sarcastic things or you might quickly become impatient with others. If you are feeling happy, you might notice yourself taking time to show caring toward a stranger or a close friend.

For your more common emotions, what cues do you notice most frequently?

When I am feeling angry, I can tell because I

_____

_____

_____

When I am feeling sad, I can tell because I

_____

_____

_____

When I am feeling happy, I can tell because I

_____

_____

_____

When I am feeling (fill in the blank) _____, I can tell because I

_____

_____

_____

How do you feel? Is that a loaded question for you? Are you able to identify how you are feeling? By now, you have become very good at logging your sexual fantasies and masturbation habits. You may have decided to take a break from masturbation and your log is pretty empty. It may also be that when you look at your log, your sexual arousal follows a pattern that is dictated by your emotions.

To examine your emotions in more detail, create an emotions log. Logs are very useful because they help us notice important patterns. What is happening with your emotions? Make notes about how you are feeling and review those notes. Use the emotions listed here to log your emotions two or three times a day. Ask yourself the following questions:

1) How Do I Feel Right Now?

It can be very hard to identify emotions, particularly if you aren't used to noticing them. If you find that identifying your emotions is very hard, keep trying. When you haven't connected with your feelings for a bit, it can seem like there is nothing there. If you think of words like neutral, ok, nothing, blank, <u>give it time and keep trying</u>. This exercise is particularly important for you!

You can also ask your friends and family to help you practice identifying your emotions. Ask them if they think you are feeling what you think you are feeling in the moment.

2) What Do I Need Right Now?

This is another very helpful question to add to your emotions log. Noticing your needs allows you to make better decisions.

Similar to your sexual fantasy log, make an emotions log that works for you. Whether you make a note on your smartphone, use an app, use one of the examples here or create your own log, it all works. A note about journaling: if you are going to journal, please ensure that you build in a schedule to review your journal in order to identify your pattern of emotions. Journals are great, but they often contain lots of information. Find a way to make it easy to retrieve the information about your emotions from your journal. You might want to make note of your main emotion in the margins of the journal; alternatively, you can underline or highlight the main emotion for each entry.

Emotions Log: Examples

Emotions Log – Template #1

Fill out each column of information

Date	Time of day	How do I feel right now? (Emotion)	What do I need right now? (Needs)	Context

Emotions Log – Template #2

Date
Emotion am:
Emotion pm:
My needs:

Date
Emotion am:
Emotion pm:
My needs:

Date
Emotion am:
Emotion pm:
My needs:

Date
Emotion am:
Emotion pm:
My needs:

> Charlie has been completing an emotions log using his cell phone for two weeks now. He is surprised to notice how often he is angry. Charlie has begun to think about why he is feeling angry so often. He realizes that he is unhappy in his relationship. Over time, he also begins to notice feelings of disappointment, sadness and rejection coming to the surface more often. He decides to find a way to fix this problem and begins to talk to his partner about attending couples' counseling together.

Anger is often identified as a secondary emotion. It is a signal that tells us that something is wrong in our lives. When you are angry, it can help to think about what is underneath the anger. For many people, it is not uncommon that anger covers a feeling of sadness or vulnerability. It can feel safer to express and feel anger rather than other emotions. Like Charlie, when you notice feelings of anger, ask yourself: **What else is going on for me right now?**

Log your emotions daily. When you review your emotion logs, what themes do you notice? Write down the main themes in the circles here.

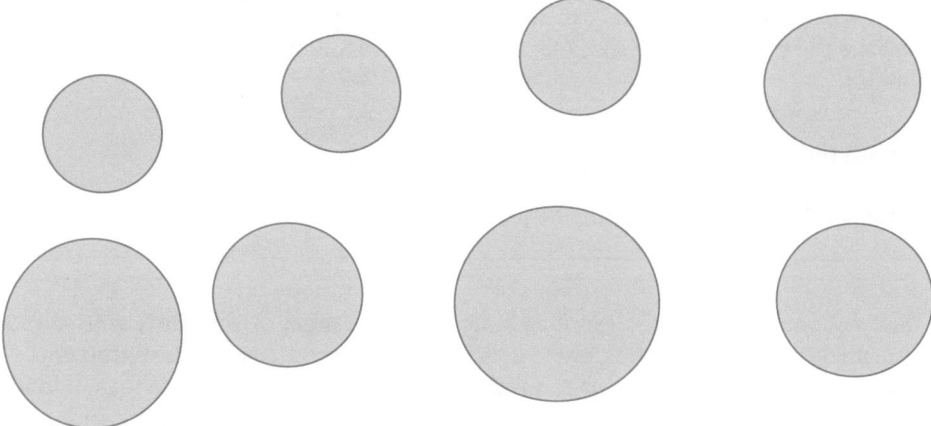

Using Sex to Feel Better

Using sex to soothe yourself or to resolve unpleasant emotions is a problem. Using sex to feel better can lead to making poor choices and poor sexual decisions. It is important to break the connection between feeling bad and having sex. Do you notice that you want to masturbate in order to deal with difficult emotions? If sex is your "go to" strategy, you are putting yourself in a very vulnerable position. When you are feeling horny or aroused, ask yourself:

How Am I Feeling Right Now? Am I Trying to Avoid a Problem or Cope With an Issue?

*Sid has not enjoyed logging his emotions. He does not like to notice his emotions. He thinks that if he does not notice his emotions, he won't feel them. It is easier to pretend that they are not there. Emotions get put away in a box, never to be addressed again. Sid has decided to ask himself an alternative question to ensure that he is not using sex to manage his emotions. Every time he feels like masturbating, he asks himself: **Am I really horny or is something else going on for me right now?** Positively, this question allows him to address his use of sex to cope with emotions without having to maintain a complicated log.*

If you are like Sid, ask yourself questions such as:

Is this a healthy situation for me?
Is this arousal a response to a difficult feeling and/or a desire to escape?
Is this a good time and a good reason to engage in sex?
Am I bored and trying to fill my time?
Am I really horny or is something else going on for me right now?

Do not move forward with sexual activity if your sexual arousal is being fueled by negative emotions. Stopping this habit may help clarify the role of emotions in your sex life. Give it a try!

A quick note about positive emotions: sometimes, positive emotions can trigger a need for sex. Positive emotions can also be used to justify behaviors. If sex is a way to celebrate situations in your life, this can also be problematic.

Robert works hard all week long. On Friday nights, it is his time to do whatever he wants. He uses this time to watch pornography and celebrate the end of the work week. Robert notices that feelings of relief, relaxation and happiness are related to his use of masturbation and sex.

Linking sex to positive emotions can lead to justifying your decision to engage in sexual activity. Take the time to notice the role of both positive and negative emotions in your life.

Notice these feelings:

SAD + LONELY + HORNY

If "Sad + Lonely + Horny" describes your emotions most of the time, your difficulties may be related to difficulties adjusting to life's various losses, challenges and problems. When this group of emotions is present, it can feel like you are in a deep pit. Feelings of loneliness amplify your sadness. Feeling sad and hopeless are problems that need to be addressed. We will discuss loneliness and the need for positive relationships in a later chapter, but for now, notice how you feel when you are surrounded by others and how you feel when you are alone. If you are sad, this may be happening for many reasons. Sometimes you are experiencing the consequences of your use of CSEM, sometimes you have unresolved problems or maybe you have suffered many losses in your life. There can be other reasons to explain your low mood. If you suspect that you are depressed, talk with your treatment provider and/or seek out your local mental health services for additional assistance.

Anxiety is an emotion that involves anticipating a threat or a danger that isn't actually in front of us. When we anticipate problems or dangers, we tend to worry a lot. For example, being afraid that someone will criticize your work and thinking that this would be terrible. Anxiety and worry can get in the way of allowing you to try new things. This can paralyze you and leave you feeling stuck. If you are feeling anxious and have many excuses not to resolve problems, not to go out and try new things, not to meet new people, not to work, etc., your anxiety might be getting in the way. Are your worries keeping you from living your fullest life? If so, talk to your treatment provider for assistance.

There are many ways to improve your emotion management skills. Notice the word *skills*. These are habits that you can practice, like other things in your life. It takes practice to improve.

Tools to improve your emotions management include:

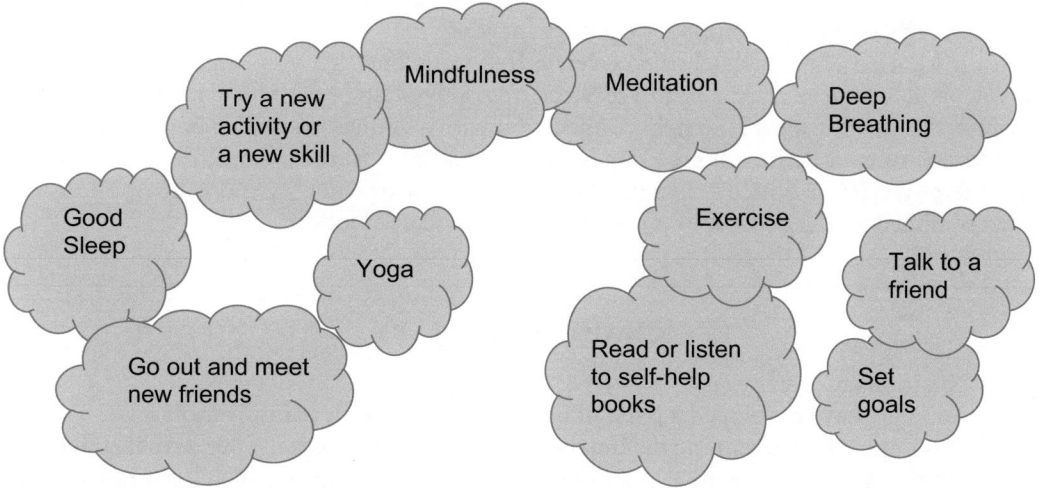

Deep breathing is a great way to calm anxiety and reduce anger. Often when we are anxious or angry, we take quick shallow breaths. Shallow breathing can worsen your negative feelings. In contrast, breathing deeply and slowly from the belly (rather than the upper chest) helps to calm us and clarify our thoughts. There are many different strategies to improve your breathing. Practice deep breathing and see how this improves your emotional state.

Another helpful skill requires practicing grounding exercises. There are many different types of grounding exercises available. Grounding exercises involve bringing yourself into the present moment. For example, ask yourself: What am I hearing? What am I seeing? What am I touching? What am I smelling? What am I tasting? Work your way through your senses while breathing deeply. Grounding exercises can help you regain your composure and help you better assess how to respond to a given situation, particularly when you are feeling emotionally heightened.

Visualization can also be very helpful. Think about a place that tends to relax you. For many people, thinking about being on a beach, hearing the waves, and smelling the saltwater can be very relaxing. For others, it might be a forest setting, hearing the wind in the trees and a gurgling river nearby. Another example might be a campfire or a candle flame. Whatever brings you peace, visualize that image. Imagine being there. Imagine what you would see, the smell and how your body would feel being there. This exercise can allow you to feel some relief from your bodily sensations of agitation, tension and fear.

Interestingly, one of the best strategies that you can use to manage your emotions is exercise. Physical exercise, particularly cardiovascular exercise, is a great way to cope with unpleasant emotions, boost mood and decrease anxiety. Exercise is as effective as or even more effective than taking anti-depressant medication.[1] Physical movement is a great way to manage intense feelings.

Once you have calmed your body, it is important to manage the thoughts that are linked to your feelings. As discussed in Chapter 4, noticing and changing unhelpful thoughts is a good way to better manage emotional states. Along with the strategies we discussed in this workbook to address your emotions management, there are some great resources available in print or in audio format. For ideas of useful self-help books, please see the list in the Recommended readings of this workbook. In addition, there are many helpful emotions management strategies available online such as breathing apps, meditation apps, mindfulness apps and emotions management apps, to name but a few. Talk to your treatment provider and reach out for additional help if you need it!

Your local community likely also offers a free crisis line that you can access 24 hours/7 days a week to receive mental health services. Your physician or your local mental health service may be good resources to help connect you with a clinical counselor in the community in addition to your treatment provider. Seeking out additional mental health services may be helpful for you if you notice a clear link between your use of sexuality and your emotions and you continue to struggle in your efforts to cope with your emotions.

CHAPTER SUMMARY

- Emotions matter!
- You may have developed a habit of using sex to deal with painful emotions.
- It is important to examine the link between your emotions and your sexual activity. Both positive and negative emotions can be linked to your sexual behaviors.
- Do not move forward with sexual activity if your sexual arousal is fueled by negative emotions.
- Improve how you address your feelings, including feelings of sadness, anger and anxiety.
- Address your emotion management needs proactively.

NOTE

1 Cooney, G. M., Dwan, K., Greig, C. A., Lawlor, D. A., Rimer, J., Waugh, F. R., McMurdo, M., & Mead, G. E. (2013). Exercise for depression. *Cochrane Database of Systematic Reviews*, Issue 9, Art. No.: CD004366. https://doi.org/10.1002/14651858.CD004366.pub6

Thoughts and Offending

CLINICIAN GUIDE

This chapter builds directly on the previous chapters, exploring general thinking errors as well as emotions management. The client can now start identifying and exploring their specific beliefs and thoughts related to sex with children, sexual images of children and using sexual images of children to enhance their own sexual arousal. Note that thinking errors can also be referred to as unhelpful thoughts, permission-giving thoughts or offense supportive thoughts. Challenges to thinking errors can be identified as replacement thoughts or alternative thoughts.

In this chapter, you are encouraged to actively explore the client's thinking as it relates to sexuality. There is much research identifying the importance of client cognitions as it relates to illegal sexual behaviors (Abel, Becker, & Cunningham-Rathner, 1984) and more particularly cognitions specific to CSEM users (see Kettleborough & Merdian, 2017; Merdian et al., 2020; Steel et al., 2020, 2021; Paquette & Cortoni, 2019, 2022; Paquette, Longpré, & Cortoni, 2020; Rimer, 2019 amongst others for a review of thinking errors specific to CSEM users). These various studies have identified different themes related to the thinking errors of CSEM users, which include their perceptions of the nature of harm, the uncontrollability of their sexual urges, minimization of the nature of harm committed by CSEM offenses, beliefs about the online environment, negative beliefs about the world and interpersonal relationships as well as specific beliefs about the sexualization of children. We frequently encounter thinking errors related to the denial of harm as it relates to CSEM use, thinking errors related to the Internet and the online world as well as beliefs surrounding the idea that children are akin to actors in these materials. As clients begin to explore themes specific to their own CSEM use, we encourage you to canvass various themes as it relates to your client's CSEM use.

Identifying the sexual thoughts that are specific to offending requires client openness and vulnerability. If the client is reluctant to engage in this discussion, it may be that the foundation of the therapeutic relationship has not been well established. If so, take the time to address any impediments within your therapeutic relationship. If you are facing a responsivity issue that cannot be resolved or is directly related to your client's willingness to engage in therapy, seek collegial consultation in order to explore alternative strategies to meet the client's needs.

Begin by asking the client to list the thinking errors they identify as it relates to their offending. Should the client not be able to identify their thinking errors, you may be able to offer some general examples or themes that have been reported by others in the past. Be

DOI: 10.4324/9781003388142-8

mindful that the examples identified by each client should be unique to their own situation and perspective. You can also ask the client to identify sexual thinking errors expressed by others in their lives; for example, family members, extended family members, other offenders they may have met online or other offenders they have met as part of their criminal justice interactions. These examples can help pave the way for them to start considering what beliefs they hold as it relates to their own sexuality and beliefs. In addition, it can be very helpful to understand the beliefs that are held in the client's environment. This can assist the client with establishing a more effective safety plan and address issues surrounding the cultural and environmental risk factors they may face.

Memory loss is often identified by clients as one reason why they cannot complete the specific exercises related to their thinking at the time of their offending. If this becomes a challenge in your work, encourage the client to work with beliefs that they held prior to offending. In addition, they can do the exercises focused on what they may have been thinking, allowing them to maintain some distance in exploring their sexual beliefs. Finally, you can also ask the clients to talk with family and friends to see if they noticed any unhelpful sexual beliefs or values that they expressed prior to their offending.

Learning to challenge thinking errors is the second step of this process. Challenging thinking errors simply means critically examining offense supportive thoughts and determining what, if any, evidence there is to support the thought. Alternatively, to challenge thinking errors, it can be helpful to ask the client if a particular belief is harmful to themselves or others. This strategy can be more effective than simply exploring the evidence available to address their beliefs. It is not unusual for clients to struggle with this task, and the clinician can provide additional information and input to help the client. For example, some clients have limited awareness of how children depicted in CSEM are impacted as they grow older and realize that the images of their abuse continue to be shared via the Internet. In some cases, clients note that children are smiling and conclude that the child is not being harmed. It is incumbent on the clinician to help the client examine their interpretation of non-verbal cues and to challenge their assumptions about those cues. Discussing their perception of non-verbal cues in the images can be a helpful addition to adequately challenging their thinking errors.

This chapter introduces the consequences to the victims depicted in CSEM. Exploring the consequences to the children and youths in CSEM, as well as their families and the community at large, can be an effective way to begin assisting the client to better understand the consequences to victims. Such consequences include the long-term impact of being viewed in sexual situations while being powerless to remove the online images (Gewirtz-Meydan et al., 2019). In addition, some clients minimize the harm to victims if they believe that the victim chose to post the images. Discussing the realities of impulsivity and peer pressure combined with delayed cognitive development occurring in adolescence can help the client challenge their beliefs related to the images that they are observing.

Understanding the long-term consequences to CSEM victims, including ongoing embarrassment, fear, discomfort and shame (Gewirtz-Meydan et al., 2018), and conveying these realities to the client is an important treatment goal. By giving the client the opportunity to critically explore and examine their offense supportive beliefs, they will hopefully be able to replace those thoughts with alternative thoughts that will reduce the risk of again accessing CSEM. If the client is able to sincerely challenge and replace offense supportive beliefs, they should be able to clearly articulate how their prior way of thinking was distorted and how such thoughts will necessarily be unhealthy for them in the future. Should clients struggle significantly with feelings of guilt and shame as a result of this work, focus on the fact that their new understanding will help them avoid CSEM use in the future.

Be mindful that some clients may simply wish to agree with the clinician's point of view. Find ways to ensure that debate and open discussion become an integral part of these discussions to facilitate the client examining their thinking patterns.

If a client is struggling to challenge their beliefs, exploring the negative impact of their beliefs on their own lives and the negative consequences to themselves is another way to assist the client to challenge their thinking patterns. At times, working with the client on the consequences to themselves can be a much more effective strategy to obtain both cognitive and behavioral change.

As discussed earlier, it can also be helpful to ask the client whether their social supports are likely to reinforce their offense supportive thoughts. If the client's social supports promote permission-giving thoughts and the victimization of children or women, the client will need to create an intervention plan to address this issue.

The work in this chapter can contribute to feelings of shame, guilt and discomfort for clients. It is therefore essential that you create an open and non-judgmental environment throughout this exploration.

REFERENCES

Abel, G. G., Becker, J. V., & Cunningham-Rathner, J. (1984). Complications, consent, and cognitions in sex between children and adults. *International Journal of Law and Psychiatry*, 7, 89–103. https://doi.org/10.1016/0160-2527(84)90008-6

Gewirtz-Meydan, A., Lahav, Y., Walsh, W., & Finkelhor, D. (2019). Psychopathology among adult survivors of child pornography. *Child Abuse & Neglect*, 98(104189), 1–11. https://doi.org/10.1016/j.chiabu.2019.104189

Gewirtz-Meydan, A., Walsh, W., Wolak, J., & Finkelhor, D. (2018). The complex experience of child pornography survivors. *Child Abuse & Neglect*, 80, 238–248. https://doi.org/10.1016/j.chiabu.2018.03.031

Kettleborough, D. G., & Merdian, H. L. (2017). Gateway to offending behaviour: Permission-giving thoughts of online users of child sexual exploitation material. *Journal of Sexual Aggression: An International, Interdisciplinary Forum for Research, Theory & Practice*, 23, 19–32. https://doi.org/10.1080/13552600.2016.1231852

Merdian, H. L., Perkins, D. E., Dustagheer, E., & Glorney, E. (2020). Development of a case formulation model for individuals who have viewed, distributed, and/ or shared child sexual exploitation material international. *Journal of Offender Therapy and Comparative Criminology*, 64(10–11), 1055–1073.

Paquette, S., & Cortoni, F. (2019). The development and validation of the Cognitions of Internet Sexual Offending (C-ISO) scale. *Sexual Abuse A Journal of Research and Treatment*, 32(8), 907–930.

Paquette, S., & Cortoni, F. (2022). Offense-supportive cognitions expressed by men who use Internet to sexually exploit children: A thematic analysis. *International Journal of Offender Therapy and Comparative Criminology*, 66(6–7), 647–669. https://doi.org/10.1177/0306624X20905757

Paquette, S., Longpré, N., & Cortoni, F. (2020). A billion distorted thoughts: An exploratory study of criminogenic cognitions among men who sexually exploit children over the Internet. *International Journal of Offender Therapy and Comparative Criminology*, 64(10–11), 1114–1133.

Rimer, J. R. (2019). "In the street they're real, in a picture they're not": Constructions of children and childhood among users of online child sexual exploitation material. *Child Abuse & Neglect*, 90, 160–173. https://doi.org/10.1016/j.chiabu.2018.12.008

Steel, C. M. S., Newman, E., O'Rourke, S., & Quayle, E. (2020). A systematic review of cognitive distortions in online child sexual exploitation material offenders. *Aggression and Violent Behavior*, 51, 101375. ISSN 1359–1789. https://doi.org/10.1016/j.avb.2020.101375

Steel, C. M. S., Newman, E., O'Rourke, S., & Quayle, E. (2021). Self perceptions and cognitions of child sexual exploitation material offenders. *International Journal of Offender Therapy and Comparative Criminology*. https://doi.org/10.1177/0306624X211062161

CLIENT WORKBOOK

Learning Objectives

In this chapter, you will:

a) learn how thoughts can lead to viewing CSEM
b) learn how thoughts can lead to a sexual offense against a child or an underage youth
c) learn how you can change your thoughts

In Chapter 4, we discussed how thinking can influence emotions and behavior. Previously, we used the term *thinking errors* or *unhelpful thoughts*. At times, we also call these "permission-giving thoughts". We have discussed the impact that thinking can have on a person's general ability to cope. We also have briefly touched on how thinking can influence offending behavior, such as accessing CSEM or the contact sexual abuse of a child or underage youth. In this chapter, we will continue to examine the link between your thoughts and your decision to access and view CSEM. Permission-giving thoughts help us step over the line and can lead to illegal behaviors. Since some who view CSEM are also interested in direct sexual contact with a child or underage youth, we will also examine thoughts that can make it easier to step in that direction.

The Connection Between Thoughts and Viewing CSEM

When we discussed the connection between thoughts, feelings, and behavior in Chapter 4, it was our hope that you would begin to examine your thinking and how it affects you. In order to understand and address what led you to access CSEM, it is necessary that you identify the thoughts that specifically led you to access CSEM. Some people may feel lonely and have thoughts about wanting to feel connected to others, but those thoughts do not necessarily lead them to access CSEM. You need to dig down and determine the specific thoughts that led you to access CSEM, as opposed to adult pornography, having a one-night stand with an adult or some other behavior. Permission-giving thoughts are what you told yourself to make it ok to offend. Identifying the thoughts that indirectly and directly led you to access CSEM can be challenging. Some people think about accessing CSEM for months or years before they actually take that step. Others may only have thoughts about accessing CSEM for a few hours or a few minutes before doing so. In either case, there were permission-giving thoughts that influenced your decision and made it easier to offend.

How long did you think of accessing CSEM before you actually did?

_____

_____

_____

_____

Identify the thoughts you had when you first decided to view CSEM. What helped you step over the line?

1) _____

_____

2) _____

_____

3) _____

_____

4) _____

_____

5) _____

_____

6) _____

_____

7) _____

_____

What thoughts helped you maintain your use of CSEM over time? What were your permission-giving thoughts?

1) _____

_____

2) _____

_____

3) _____

_____

4) _____

_____

5) _____

_____

6) _____

_____

7) _____

_____

If you are struggling to identify your thoughts, here you will see a number of thoughts that have been found to facilitate the viewing of CSEM. Which of the following can be added to the thoughts that you have already identified? Underline those that apply to you.

General Thoughts	Permission-Giving Thoughts
Thoughts about children and underage youth	– If a child or underage youth talks to me about sex online, it means they want to have sex. – The children or underage youths in CSEM are not like those in real life. – The children or underage youths in CSEM are sexually seductive. – The children or underage youths in CSEM who smile clearly are enjoying what they are doing. – Children or underage youths are sexually attractive. – The innocence and beauty of children or underage youths attracts me to CSEM. – Viewing images of sexually developed teens is different from viewing undeveloped children. – Children or underage youths who post images of themselves masturbating or engaged in sex with a peer don't care who looks at the images.
Thoughts about yourself	– I enjoy collecting and organizing CSEM. – CSEM helps me feel better when I feel sad/lonely/bored/angry. – CSEM gives me a sense of excitement. – I like breaking rules, and CSEM is a way to do that. – I should be able to do what I want – even if others don't like it. – I can't control myself when I see CSEM. – Viewing CSEM provides me with a sense that I am part of a community. – Viewing CSEM gives me a sense of power.
Thoughts about the Internet	– The Internet is a safe place to do things I would not do in real life. – The Internet allows me to escape reality. – Rather than being rejected in the offline world, the Internet allows me to have conversations with others. – The Internet is not real – it is just fantasy. – The Internet is a private space for me. – Lots of people on the Internet look at CSEM. – The accessibility of CSEM on the Internet means it's okay to look at. – On the Internet, it is easy to lose control when browsing.

Thoughts about the impact of CSEM	– If I am just watching CSEM, I am not actually hurting anyone. – If no one knows that I am viewing CSEM, then no one is hurt. – Sexually developed teens who are in CSEM are not harmed. – Viewing CSEM is not even close to being as bad as actually sexually touching a child or underage youth. – Society should be happy that men look at CSEM rather than actually sexually abuse children or underage youths. – CSEM is a good way to keep men from sexually abusing children and underage youths.
Thoughts about your sexual interests and sexuality	– My interest in sexual materials such as bestiality or hentai led me to view CSEM, the more unusual the better. – A general interest in extreme sexual behavior rather than a sexual interest in children or underage youths led me to view CSEM. – I have such a high sex drive that anything sexual will turn me on, CSEM was just the latest thing. – I have a sexual addiction and CSEM is just part of that.

Are there additional thoughts that may have influenced your decision to view CSEM? People often have to keep digging to identify the thoughts that influenced their decision to view CSEM. Go ahead and list the additional thoughts that apply to you.

8) _____

_____

9) _____

_____

10) _____

_____

11) _____

_____

12) _____

_____

13) _____

_____

14) _____

_____

15) _____

_____

The Connection Between Thoughts and Contact Sexual Offending of a Child or Underage Youth

Although research suggests that few men who are arrested for viewing CSEM later commit a contact offense against a child or underage youth, there are some who do. Some men also communicate with children or underage youth online via live webcams and directly interact sexually with a child or underage youth. As such, it is important to discuss some of the thoughts that can make you more vulnerable to a contact offense against a child or underage youth, as well as thoughts that can lead to using the Internet to directly communicate and interact sexually with a child. To help you with this task, review the thoughts described here. You will notice some overlap with the themes that you reviewed earlier. Underline those that apply to you.

Topics	Permission-Giving Thoughts
Children and underage youths	– Some children or underage youth are mature enough to enjoy sex with an adult. – If a child or underage youth does not say "no" to engaging sexually with an adult, it means the child wants to have sex. – Children or underage youths are often able to understand an adult's sexual needs. – Children or underage youths are sexually provocative. – The innocence and beauty of children or underage youths sexually attracts me. – Children or underage youths really listen to me. – Children or underage youths like chatting about sex on the Internet with adults. – Children or underage youths really like me and want to be sexual with me.
The world	– Society is too uptight about sex between children or underage youths and adults. – I won't let society control what I do. – Society tries to stop me from having the life I deserve. – I have never gotten a fair deal from others, so I can take what I want, whether it be sex or anything else. – After being pushed down for so long, it is only fair that I push back.

Yourself	– I have more in common with children or underage youths than other adults. – I am capable of falling in love with a child or underage youth. – I am happier when I am sexual with a child or an underage youth. – Online sexual chatting with a child or underage youth excites me. – I feel emotionally safer and more accepted by children or underage youths.
The impact of adult and child sexual activity	– My relationship with my son or daughter is strengthened by having sex together. – If a child or underage youth has sex with an adult, she or he will look back and see it as a positive experience. – Sex between a child or underage youth and an adult helps teach him or her about sex. – Sex between a child or underage youth and an adult helps teach him or her about love. – Simply chatting online about sex with a child or underage youth does not do any harm. – It is okay to arrange to meet a child or underage youth for sex if she or he is willing.
Sex and sexuality	– If I go without sex, I suffer. – I am entitled to sex. – Men need more sex than women do. – I have such a high sex drive that anything sexual will turn me on, including sex with a child or underage youth. – I have such a high sex drive that when the urge begins, I can't stop it. – I have a sexual addiction and that is why I fantasize about having sex with a child or underage youth.

With which of these thoughts do you agree? List them.

1) _____

_____

2) _____

_____

3) _____

_____

4) _____

_____

5) _____

_____

6) _____

_____

7) _____

_____

8) _____

_____

How Can You Change Your Thoughts?

If you wish to have a healthy life where you are less vulnerable to viewing CSEM and less vulnerable to committing a contact offense against a child or underage youth, then you will need to carefully examine the thoughts that applied to you. As in Chapter 4, we encourage you to challenge your thinking. Are the permission-giving thoughts that helped you to step over the line facts or opinions? Where is the evidence? Are the permission-giving thoughts helpful to you and your goals in life?

For example, where is the evidence that children are capable of deciding to engage in online sexual behavior or are capable of deciding to be sexual with an adult? The reality is that children and underage youths are not able to legally consent to sexual activity. They cannot legally consent to making sexual images. This is likely most readily understood in regard to images, where it is clear that a child is being forcefully sexually abused. Other times, youths under 18 may not appear to be in distress or they may even appear to be enjoying the experience. However, there are many reasons this might be the case. Sometimes victims were tricked into taking the images; sometimes they feel forced to take the images to obtain money or social privileges; and sometimes the image was taken to send to a specific person but was posted elsewhere without the victim's consent. Of course, even in cases where youths post images of themselves masturbating, they lack the maturity and understanding of the long-term consequences of such acts. In fact, victims often speak about the fear of being recognized by strangers who have seen their images – even long after the images were created. You are one of those people they fear may recognize them. Victims report significant distress, shame and negative consequences in their own lives and in their mental health as a result of their images being online. Victims note that the images are a shameful reminder of their abuse, of their victimization by others or of their willingness to post images that led to marked feelings of vulnerability and regret. *This is not a victimless crime.*

The victims in the pictures are affected by the fact that their images are online and by the fact that others are viewing their images for sexual arousal. Victims are harmed by this ongoing abuse. There is ongoing, continual abuse when your image is being used for a sexual purpose without your consent. Victims are affected by their lack of control about who is viewing their images. Victims are harmed by ongoing fear, shame and anger and report fearing being judged by others because their images are being circulated online. So, is it really true that by "just looking" at CSEM, you are doing no harm?

Let's reflect further on the impact on victims. Victims of sexual abuse report experiencing many different consequences. They report difficulty with intimacy, difficulty with trust, increased use of drugs or alcohol to cope, limiting their social interactions for fear of being detected, fear of establishing a new relationship due to the need to disclose this fact to the new partner, increased anxiety, depression, and changes in how they view their bodies, increased social isolation, ongoing shame, loss of self-worth, suicidal ideation and many other negative consequences. Victims report consequences for their loved ones, who watch them struggle and who may feel guilty about their inability to protect the victim from harm. Of course, part of the reason the images were made in the first place is because adult sexual abusers know there is a market for such images – and that motivates them to abuse children and to make images of that abuse. So, again, is it really true that by "just looking" at CSEM you are doing no harm?

Of course, the nature of the Internet can make it more difficult to realize that the children in CSEM are real children. Perhaps you were able to distance yourself emotionally from that reality. If you witnessed what you saw on your computer or cell phone through a window as you were walking home, would you have more concern for the child?[1] If the children depicted in CSEM are from overseas or have a skin color that is different from yours, does that make their experience any less painful or harmful? Is it possible that the children in CSEM are just like the kids in your community? It helps to remember that these are not "just" images – they are people.

Communities react very strongly to sexual offenses against children and youths. People talk negatively about sexual crimes. Community concerns are heightened every time sexual offenses are reported. Communities shun strangers and try to keep their children safe in an effort to keep them from being victims of sexual crimes. In addition, we spend significant time, money and tax dollars to pay for the criminal justice interventions required to manage sexual crimes (for example, police investigations, court system, judicial system, etc.). Each time you view CSEM, it has an impact on the entire community. It spreads fear and concern and heightens the need for vigilance in others.

Let's review. Answer these questions.

How are the children and underage youths depicted in CSEM negatively impacted?

_____

_____

_____

_____

_____

How are the parents of the children and youths depicted in CSEM negatively impacted?

_____

_____

_____

_____

How are the families, friends and loved ones of the children and youths depicted in CSEM negatively impacted?

_____

_____

_____

_____

How is the community negatively impacted by the use of CSEM?

_____

_____

_____

_____

In this exercise, identify each of the permission-giving thoughts that made you more vulnerable to viewing CSEM. Then, challenge that thought by asking yourself what evidence you have for and against that thought. If you wish to truly rid yourself of the thoughts that increase your risk of future CSEM use or contact offense against a child or underage youth, what is the best and most convincing replacement thought?

1) My thought

_____

_____

Challenge the thought. Fact or opinion? Will this thought do harm?

_____

_____

_____

_____

_____

My replacement thought

_____

_____

_____

_____

_____

2) My thought

_____

_____

Challenge the thought. Fact or opinion? Will this thought do harm?

_____

_____

_____

_____

_____

My replacement thought

_____

_____

_____

_____

3) My thought

_____

_____

Challenge the thought. Fact or opinion? Will this thought do harm?

_____

_____

_____

_____

_____

My replacement thought

_____

_____

_____

_____

4) My thought

_____

_____

Challenge the thought. Fact or opinion? Will this thought do harm?

_____

_____

_____

_____

_____

My replacement thought

_____

_____

_____

_____

_____

5) My thought

_____

_____

Challenge the thought. Fact or opinion? Will this thought do harm?

_____

_____

_____

_____

My replacement thought

_____

_____

_____

_____

6) My thought

_____

_____

Challenge the thought. Fact or opinion? Will this thought do harm?

_____

_____

_____

_____

_____

My replacement thought

_____

_____

_____

_____

7) My thought

_____

_____

Challenge the thought. Fact or opinion? Will this thought do harm?

_____

_____

_____

_____

_____

My replacement thought

_____

_____

_____

_____

8) My thought

_____

_____

Challenge the thought. Fact or opinion? Will this thought do harm?

_____

_____

_____

_____

_____

My replacement thought

_____

_____

_____

_____

_____

Continue this work on a separate piece of paper as needed.

Challenging and replacing your thoughts can be difficult. Indeed, sometimes it is very difficult to see our own blind spots. Ask someone you trust to review your challenges and replacement thoughts. Do they make sense to that person? Discussing your work with your therapist is essential.

If you struggled to develop replacement thoughts that you find truly convincing, it will be even more important for you to seek help. Fortunately, if you were willing to work on identifying your offense-supportive thoughts, then you have already taken an important step forward. Keep working at it!

The next chapter addresses additional sexual issues and other factors that contributed to your accessing and viewing CSEM.

CHAPTER SUMMARY

- In order to help ensure a healthy life that does not include further viewing of CSEM, it is essential that you identify the thoughts that made it easier for you to view and to keep viewing CSEM.
- Given that some men are also interested in sexual contact with a child, it is also important that you identify any thoughts that make you more vulnerable to such an offense.
- Victims are negatively impacted by your CSEM use. There are many negative consequences for victims of CSEM.
- Once you have identified the unhelpful thoughts related to your use of CSEM, you need to challenge those thoughts and develop replacement thoughts that are truly convincing for you.
- It is often helpful to find a trusted person who can help you critically evaluate your challenges and your replacement thoughts.

NOTE

1   Rimer, J. R. (2019). "In the street they're real, in a picture they're not": Constructions of children and childhood among users of online child sexual exploitation material. *Child Abuse & Neglect*, *90*, 160–173. https://doi.org/10.1016/j.chiabu.2018.12.008

8

Sexual Management: Advanced Topics

CLINICIAN GUIDE

In this chapter, we explore more detailed topics related to sexuality. It is now the time to ensure that sexual issues you haven't reviewed or discussed are explored in more detail. Before starting this work, take the time to review your treatment plan and session notes. Identify gaps in your knowledge about the client's sexuality, sexual arousal patterns, sexual history, use of sex to cope, sexual preoccupation, sexual preferences and sexual interests. Make note of sexual themes and issues that have not yet been addressed. In addition, we also encourage you to review any current risks to children in the community. Ensure that the client has not developed new relationships that involve children and that there are no new children who have entered their lives. Overall, it is a good time to ensure that you are clear about what sexual topics remain to be explored to effectively manage the client's sexuality and their sexual urges.

We start by reviewing sexual consent. Identify the importance of verbal consent, discuss enthusiastic consent and the pitfalls related to relying on non-verbal cues to obtain consent. Often, elements of sexual consent are not very clear for clients. Clearly knowing who can and cannot consent is fundamental knowledge for the client to understand. There are many online resources to help you address consent. Although it's not specific to CSEM, a popular YouTube video entitled Sex and Tea uses a humorous approach to examine this fundamental issue. Discussing consent by breaking down enthusiastic consent, willing consent, unwilling consent and coerced consent can also be a useful framework (see Chen, 2020 and Nagoski, 2022 for details).

If you have not done so already, this is the time to discuss pedophilia/hebephilia. It is important to discuss sexual attraction to children openly. For some clients, it can be important to review the research that has found a link between biological factors and pedophilia. This can help reduce shame. There are many studies examining the biological underpinnings of pedophilia, and you are encouraged to ensure that you have an understanding of the theories related to pedophilia (see Dyshniku et al., 2015; Fazio et al., 2017; Seto, 2018, 2017, 2013, 2012 for details).

You want to know when thoughts related to children began and the frequency and regularity of such thoughts over time. Some key questions may be:

- Were they themselves abused as children?
- What is it about children that they find appealing?

DOI: 10.4324/9781003388142-9

- Are they attracted to innocence or to the process of puberty?
- Are they attracted to the skin texture of children?
- Do they find children more accepting?
- Did they experience sexual interactions as children?
- Did they experience sexual interactions with same sex or opposite sex as children/youths?
- At what age did they first see CSEM?

For some clients, the main draw is the power that they ultimately have over children, particularly when they do not experience this power in their same-age relationships. Exploring these themes from a non-judgmental perspective and discussing the nature of their sexual interests will help clients create an efficient safety plan.

It is recommended that for pedophilic or hebephilic clients, you work collaboratively to encourage and enhance a sexual interest in adults. Create an arousal management plan that focuses on adult sexual thoughts and fantasies. Encourage your clients to explore all the aspects of sexuality with consensual adult partners. This is an important treatment target. Work with a therapist who has experience working with men who have committed sexually motivated offenses to increase your knowledge of strategies to create effective arousal management plans, if this is not your current area of expertise.

Adult pornography is also addressed in this chapter. This can be a controversial issue. Research has not yet addressed this issue in any depth for those who have accessed CSEM. Individual differences have been found to play a significant mediating role on the impact of pornography use for men who have committed sexual offenses (Saramago, Cardoso, & Lea, 2019; Malamuth, Hald, & Koss, 2012; Fisher et al., 2013; Kingston et al., 2008, 2009; Seto, Maric, & Barbaree, 2001). There is also a thoughtful investigation on the impact of personal beliefs and attitudes about whether pornography is problematic for offenders (Mellor & Duff, 2019). Whether or not a person views pornography use as a concern is an essential consideration for any clinician.

Holt et al. (2021) conducted research with men who were convicted of sexual offenses and examined their views of pornography in their offending and future functioning. These results suggest that the following themes may be informative when clinicians are discussing the role that pornography has in their clients' lives: pornography as a consumption problem (addictions, problematic consumption); pornography as a facilitation problem (impacting personal values, facilitating offending due to the impact on beliefs, attitudes and thinking errors); pornography as inhibiting (not impacting risk, not related to offending or used to inhibit offending) and learning control (pornography as a way to learn control, establishing healthy pornography practices) (please see Holt et al., 2021 for details). Clinicians may find it helpful to utilize a screening tool such as the Pornography Consumption Effects Scale to explore this issue in more detail (see Miller, Kidd, & Hald, 2019; Miller, Hald, & Kidd, 2018; Hald & Malamuth, 2008 for details).

As clearly indicated in the research literature, not everyone who accesses pornography experiences problems as a result. For many people, the use of pornography can be a part of a satisfying sexual experience, and many find that this enhances their sexual life when used carefully and thoughtfully; however, there are some individuals for whom pornography use is clearly problematic. Despite this fact, clients will likely have access to adult pornography at some point in their lives. Many clients may also wish to continue using adult pornography. Whether or not your work environment permits clients to use adult pornography, this topic remains relevant to discuss. The clinician's challenge is to explore this issue in a curious and non-judgmental manner so that the client can ultimately make an informed and healthy choice.

There are many details about the client's use of adult pornography that are helpful to discuss. In addition to the questions identified in the client's workbook section of this chapter, some additional questions to consider may include:

- When do they use pornography?
- What type of adult pornography do they enjoy?
- Where do they access adult pornography?
- How do they access adult pornography, using what type of device?
- How did their past pornography use contribute to their offending?
- How did their past pornography use impact their beliefs about sexuality and/or relationships?
- What are their concerns about any future risk related to their use of pornography?
- Would they like to include adult pornography in their lives?
- What are their beliefs about various sources of ethical adult pornography?
- Will they continue to use pornography?

We understand that some clinicians may be prone to unilaterally prohibiting CSEM clients from accessing adult pornography. We believe that asking the client to identify their intentions using an open and client-centered approach enhances the therapeutic relationship and ultimately facilitates an improved therapeutic discussion about the pros and cons of the client's desire to access or not access adult pornography. Ultimately, clients will make their own decisions about this issue. Best practices would suggest that it is the clinician's role to facilitate a thoughtful consideration of that choice, rather than to make the choice for the client.

Discussing issues related to sexual performance is essential. In our clinical experience, CSEM offenders often present with concerns related to their sexual performance. Frequently, clients report sexual issues such as erection problems, ejaculation problems, difficulties with desire and/or concerns about their genitalia. Of note, people who are diagnosed with ADHD present with higher rates of sexual dysfunctions (Soldati et al., 2020; Bijlenga et al., 2018). Sexual performance issues are important to address because if clients are not comfortable or successful in partnered sexual activities for whatever reason, their tendency to drift online to fulfill their sexual needs will likely increase.

There are different realities involved in partnered sex vs solo sex. Partnered sex requires relationship skills, negotiation and compromise. Solo sex allows people to focus solely on their own needs, wants, pleasure and personal requirements. This is an important distinction, and we encourage you to discuss it within this module. Some relevant questions include:

- What is your client's preference as it relates to either partnered or solo sex?
- Has their preference been mostly achieved in their lives?
- What are the barriers to achieving partnered sex?
- If they prefer solo sex, how will this be better managed moving forward?

In addition, it is important to address gender issues and sexual orientation. Ensure that you do not make any assumptions about their sexual orientation or their gender. Past sexual choices, sexual activities and/or current gender presentations do not necessarily reflect their sexual orientation or the presence of gender issues. This is particularly problematic in communities where LGBTQ+ choices are not valued, not safe and/or are not openly acknowledged. It may be that clients have not admitted to themselves, much less to others, that their past choices do not reflect their sexual orientation or preferred gender. Take the time to discuss gender issues and sexual preferences. Allow the client to reflect on these issues and to consider their patterns of arousal. Encourage clients to openly discuss any questions they have about their gender and sexual orientation. Ensure that the therapeutic environment allows for the safe expression and safe discussion of these important themes.

Both you and the client should feel that sexuality is well understood and managed by the end of this chapter. If that is not the case, it will be important to go back and see what might be missing in the understanding and application of the client's sexual risk factors. If you believe that your client requires additional assistance to manage their sexual urges, sexual interests and/or sexual behaviors, now is the time to ensure that you have a psychiatrist or physician actively working with you as part of the client's treatment plan. Referrals for pharmacological interventions to help address sexual risk should be implemented if it is relevant for your client.

This is also a good time to ensure that you engage in professional consultation to see if there are any issues that you have not addressed or identified which are relevant for your client's treatment plan prior to moving on to the next chapters, which examine their relationships and their use of the Internet. The goal of building effective safety plans with the client requires fully addressing their sexual needs and concerns. If you are not confident about how the sexual risk factors have been addressed with your client, seek professional consultation to discuss the client's needs in more detail.

REFERENCES

Bijlenga, D., Vroege, J. A., Stammen, A. J. M., et al. (2018). Prevalence of sexual dysfunctions and other sexual disorders in adults with attention-deficit/hyperactivity disorder compared to the general population. *ADHD Attention Deficit Hyperactivity Disorders, 10*, 87–96.

Chen, A. (2020). *Ace: What asexuality reveals about desire, society, and the meaning of sex*. Boston: Beacon Press.

Dyshniku, F., Murray, M. E., Fazio, R. L., Lykins, A. D., & Cantor, J. M. (2015). Minor physical anomalies as a window into the prenatal origins of pedophilia. *Archives of Sexual Behavior, 44*, 2151–2159. https://doi.org/10.1007/s10508-015-0564-7

Fazio, R. L., Dyshniku, F., Lykins, A. D., & Cantor, J. M. (2017). Leg length versus torso length in pedophilia: Further evidence of atypical physical development early in life. *Sexual Abuse: Journal of Research and Treatment, 29*, 500–514.

Fisher, W. A., Kohut, T., Di Gioacchino, L. A., & Fedoroff, P. (2013). Pornography, sex crime, and paraphilia. *Current Psychiatry Reports, 15*, 362. https://doi.org/10.1007/s11920-013-0362-7

Hald, G. M., & Malamuth, N. M. (2008). Self-perceived effects of pornography consumption. *Archives of Sexual Behavior, 37*(4), 614–625.

Holt, K., Kissinger, J., Spickler, C., & Roush, V. (2021). Pornography use and sexual offending: An examination of perceptions of role and risk. *International Journal of Offender Therapy and Comparative Criminology*, 1–25. https://doi.org/10.1177/0306624X211049183

Kingston, D. A., Fedoroff, P., Firestone, P., Curry, S., & Bradford, J. M. (2008). Pornography use and sexual aggression: The impact of frequency and type of pornography use on recidivism among sexual offenders. *Aggressive Behavior, 34*, 1–11.

Kingston, D. A., Malamuth, N. M., Fedoroff, P., & Marshall, W. L. (2009). The importance of individual differences in pornography use: Theoretical perspectives and implications for treating sexual offenders. *The Journal of Sex Research, 46*(2/3), 216–232. www.jstor.org/stable/20620415

Malamuth, N. M., Hald, G. M., & Koss, M. (2012). Pornography, individual differences in risk and men's acceptance of violence against women in a representative sample. *Sex Roles, 66*(7–8), 427–439.

Mellor, E., & Duff, S. (2019). A quantitative analysis of attitudes toward pornography use in secure hospitals: Sexual, violent and non-offenders [Attitudes toward pornography use]. *Journal of Forensic Practice, 21*(2), 112–123. https://doi.org/10.1108/JFP-12-2018-0049

Miller, D. J., Hald, G. M., & Kidd, G. (2018). Self-perceived effects of pornography consumption among heterosexual men. *Psychology of Men & Masculinity, 19*(3), 469–476. http://doi.org/10.1037/men0000112

Miller, D. J., Kidd, G., & Hald, G. M. (2019). Measuring self-perceived effects of pornography: A short-form version of the pornography consumption effects scale. *Archives of Sexual Behavior, 48*, 753–761. https://doi.org/10.1007/s10508-018-1327-z

Nagoski, E. (2022, April). Enthusiastic, willing, unwilling, coerced: Consent, in the context of sex worth having. *Confidence & Joy Newsletter*. https://emilynagoski.bulletin.com/enthusiastic-willing-unwilling-coerced/

Saramago, M. A., Cardoso, J., & Lea, I. (2019). Pornography use by sex offenders at the time of the index offense: Characterization and predictors. *Journal of Sex and Marital Therapy, 45*(6), 473–487.

Seto, M. C. (2012). Is pedophilia a sexual orientation? *Archives of Sexual Behavior, 41*(1), 231–236.

Seto, M. C. (2013). *Internet sex offenders*. Washington, DC: APA Books.

Seto, M. C. (2017). The puzzle of male chronophilias. *Archives of Sexual Behavavior, 46*, 3–22. https://doi.org/10.1007/s10508-016-0799-y

Seto, M. C. (2018). *Pedophilia and sexual offending against children: Theory, assessment, and intervention* (2nd ed.). Washington, DC: APA Books.

Seto, M. C., Maric, A. M., & Barbaree, H. E. (2001). The role of pornography in the etiology of sexual aggression. *Aggression and Violent Behavior, 6*(1), 35–53. https://doi.org/10.1016/S1359-1789(99)00007-5

Soldati, L., Bianchi-Demicheli, F., Schockaert, P., Köhl, J., Bolmont, M., Hasler, R., & Perroud, N. (2020). Sexual function, sexual dysfunctions, and ADHD: A systematic literature review. *Journal of Sexual Medicine, 17*(9), 1653. https://doi.org/10.1016/j.jsxm.2020.03.019

CLIENT WORKBOOK

Learning Objectives

In this chapter, you will:

a) learn about the rules of sexual consent
b) reflect on the topic of sexual interest in children
c) reflect on your use of adult pornography
d) reflect on the impact of sexual performance issues
e) reflect on gender identity and sexual orientation

In this chapter, we will be addressing more advanced topics related to sexual management. The first topic is sexual consent. Let's start with the rules of sexual consent. While this may seem obvious to you, there are rules about sex. There are rules about what is legal and what is illegal. Sometimes the rules aren't clear, the rules change or the rules don't make sense to you. It is essential that you follow the rules in your country/state/province/territory or municipality. Whatever form your legal system takes, please defer to your local rules.

• What are the rules in your local area?
• What sexual behaviors can result in your arrest?
• What are the legal consequences when you get caught?

Look up the local laws about sex in your area. You will likely find this information by searching online for "Sexual laws in XX" (fill in your country/province/state/territory). What did you find? What is allowed? What is not allowed?

_____

_____

_____

_____

Now explore the consequences for breaching these laws. What are the penalties? What are the typical sentence lengths? What are the typical prison sentences? What are the typical community supervision sentences?

_____

_____

_____

_____

We expect that you may have been surprised by the rules of consent, as well as the penalties involved in breaching these rules in your jurisdiction. There are specific ages associated with consent and sexual activity. There are rules about sex with people when you hold a position of power in the relationship such as a teacher, counsellor, babysitter, employer or other authority figure. It is important to know and follow the rules, regardless of how you feel about these rules!

There are also rules about the conditions that would impede someone's ability to provide consent to a sexual partner. This means that if your sexual partner is intoxicated, unconscious, sleeping or not coherent, they are not able to consent to sexual activity regardless of their age. You can't have sex with someone who is not able to answer the question "Do you want to have sex with me?"

There are rules about listening to your partner. No means no. At all times in sexual situations, no means no, stop means stop and I don't know means no. If you have started to engage someone sexually and they ask you to stop, then you must stop. Even if you are in the middle of sexual intercourse, you must stop.

A note about consent: if you are with an adult partner and they have not said yes to sex, then it is best to assume that the answer is no. A good habit is to ask directly if someone wants to have sex with you. Clarity is important. Just because someone is kissing you doesn't mean that they want to have sex with you. Ask directly. Talking about sex with your partners is an important part of staying safe and ensuring that both of you are consenting to all your sexual interactions.

Sexual Attraction to Children

In Chapter 3, we discussed the features that indicate whether someone has a pedophilic interest and/or a hebephilic sexual interest. It takes a great deal of courage to acknowledge such a sexual interest, because there is a lot of stigma associated with a sexual interest in children. There can also be a lot of shame. In some cases, people confuse the presence of a sexual interest in children with the notion that someone with such an interest also necessarily sexually abuses children. We know that while some people with this interest do progress to sexually abusing a child, there are many who do not. Importantly, there is a difference between having a sexual interest in children and engaging in a contact offense against a child. Some individuals who access CSEM do so in an attempt to satisfy their sexual interest in children, in hopes that this will help prevent them from engaging in a contact offense against a child. Although the desire to avoid a contact offense against a child is commendable, it is important to remember that children are harmed by the making of CSEM and that the market for CSEM is fueled by people willing to view the images. In addition, the content of your sexual fantasies can fuel your sexual interests. For others, the use of CSEM was part of a broader interest in actually engaging in contact offenses against children. Failing to recognize and acknowledge a sexual interest in children, if it exists, leaves a large gap in your understanding of the factors that influenced your decision to access CSEM. If you have a sexual interest in children, have you been able to admit that to yourself and possibly a trusted support? If not, what are the barriers that have gotten in the way of admitting that to yourself and to trusted others?

. . . .
1   2   3   4   5

1 = Untrue of me
2 = Sometimes true of me
3 = Often true of me
4 = True of me
5 = Very true of me

1) Shame: thinking that my sexual interest in children means I am a terrible person.	1	2	3	4	5
2) Fear that others will reject me.	1	2	3	4	5
3) Fear that others will physically hurt me.	1	2	3	4	5
4) Fear that simply having such an interest means that someone will have to report me to police.	1	2	3	4	5
5) Lack of trust in my current treatment provider.	1	2	3	4	5
6) Fear that my friends or my family will abandon me.	1	2	3	4	5
7) Other: _____	1	2	3	4	5

It is important to know that a sexual interest in children is not something that someone chooses. Indeed, who would choose a sexual interest that is stigmatized and can leave one feeling separate from others and afraid to discuss such an essential aspect of themselves?

How does sexual interest in children develop? Unfortunately, we do not yet have a definitive answer to this question, but research suggests it is not an interest that someone simply chooses. For example, there is research that indicates that it may be "hardwired" in the brain. It has also been suggested that there can be a link with early childhood abuse. The mechanisms of this link are not entirely clear. However, the majority of sexually abused children do not go on to commit sexual offenses later in life. It is important to understand that a sexual interest in children is not going to go away with willpower or simply because one hopes or wishes that it will. Shame can get in the way of admitting to having a sexual interest in children. There is a difference between having an interest and acting on that interest. This understanding is important in overcoming shame.

If you have an interest in children, you are going to need to deal with that interest directly and purposefully. Fortunately, although an interest in children cannot be willed away, it can be managed. The first step is, of course, admitting the interest to yourself. The next step can involve telling someone you trust. If you do not have supports you can trust with this information, there are online support groups, such as Virtuous Pedophiles. This group provides emotional support for those who are sexually interested in children but who do not wish to act on that interest. Indeed, finding another person to whom you can turn for support is often an essential step toward feeling less lonely and less isolated – issues that often play a role in increasing one's vulnerability to acting out a sexual interest in children, either through viewing CSEM or by engaging in a contact offense against a child. Reaching out to another trusted person or persons is also often the first step to escaping the shame that some feel about their sexual interest in children. Talk with your treatment provider about safe people with whom you may want to share these concerns. Discuss the advantages and disadvantages of broadening your trusted circle of accountability. Of course, reaching out to someone and letting them know about such a personal issue can be difficult.

1) I agree that it will be helpful to let a trusted person know about my sexual interest in children. Y___/N___

    Why? _____

    _____

_____

_____

_____

2) I am ready to let a trusted person know about my sexual interest in children. Y___/N___

   Why? _____

   _____

   _____

   _____

   _____

3) If you are ready to let a trusted person know about your sexual interest in children, who will you talk to? _____

   _____

   _____

   _____

   _____

As noted elsewhere in this workbook, discuss with your treatment provider the need to seek out a psychiatrist or physician with expertise in this area, as there are also medications that can help to manage sexual fantasy and urges. If you are having marked difficulty managing your sexual fantasies of children and you are concerned you will act on your urges by accessing CSEM or by engaging in a contact sexual offense against a child, medication can be a useful intervention. However, medication alone will not be enough. It is important to develop the emotional and sexual regulation skills we have discussed throughout this workbook and to put physical barriers between you and your urges that may result in harm toward a child. This may involve moving out of a residence where there is a child you have access to, or it may mean ensuring that someone else oversees all your online activities. A small note: if you do have pedophilic or hebephilic interests, it may take time to enhance your sexual interest in adults. Discuss this goal with your treatment provider. There are many aspects to managing a sexual interest in children. If you have a sexual interest in children, what are your next steps?

1. Tell a trusted support that I need their help to manage my sexual interest in children. Y___/N___

   a. Identify what type of help you will ask for.

   _____

   _____

   _____

   _____

    b. Consult with a physician regarding medication to help manage my fantasies and urges. Y____/N____

       When? _____

    c. How will you find a physician?

_____

_____

2. Creating physical barriers between me and access to children. Y____/N____

    a. What barriers will you put in place?

_____

_____

_____

If you have already put some of these interventions in place, congratulations! If there are other needed interventions that you have yet to put into place, we encourage you to make these a priority.

Using Adult Pornography

An additional topic that deserves consideration is whether adult pornography can be safely integrated into your sexual life. This is a challenging question. Research has not yet addressed this issue in any depth for those who have accessed CSEM.

It can be helpful to consider these questions when reflecting on your past pornography use:[1]

- Was your pornography use too much, uncontrolled and/or unmanageable?
- Did you feel like your pornography use was "an addiction"?
- Did pornography influence your beliefs and attitudes about others?
- Did pornography facilitate your thinking errors or permission-giving thoughts about offending?
- Was pornography use related or unrelated to your use of CSEM?
- Do you believe that accessing adult pornography would help you avoid future CSEM use?
- Do you believe that you need assistance to learn how to better manage your pornography use in the future?

You will be required to make a decision about your pornography use, either now or in the future. An important question to consider is: what is the healthiest choice for YOU? Are you more vulnerable to falling back on CSEM use if you access adult pornography? If accessing adult images leads you to CSEM, is that a risk you are willing to take?

Other questions to consider include:

- Does your use of adult pornography distort your view of your adult sexual partner(s)?
- Does your use of adult pornography change your expectations of sex with an adult sexual partner(s)?
- Does your use of adult pornography cause distress for your current partner?

- Are you able to manage your use of adult pornography without problems?
- Does your use of adult pornography add to a satisfying sexual life, either by yourself or with your partner?
- Does adult pornography enhance your life?
- Will your use of adult pornography help you to avoid accessing CSEM?

What are the risks of accessing adult pornography for you?

1) _____

2) _____

3) _____

4) _____

What are the benefits of accessing adult pornography for you?

1) _____

2) _____

3) _____

4) _____

In the future I (check an answer):
1) __Intend to access adult pornography
2) __Intend to cease all use of adult pornography
3) __Am not sure what I want to do

Sexual Performance Concerns

Some people find that they have many concerns about their ability to please and satisfy a sexual partner. Sexual performance issues can be difficult. You may feel embarrassed about the presence of a sexual performance problem. Sexual performance problems can lead to more pornography use. In fact, if you are concerned that you cannot satisfy a sexual partner, it may feel safer to use the Internet to deal with your sexual urges. Partnered sex is a different experience than solo sex. Sometimes, it may feel simpler to address your sexual needs alone rather than with a partner. There are many potential problems with making the Internet your sexual playground. Dealing with your sexual concerns is an important step toward ceasing your CSEM use.

The need to satisfy a sexual partner can feel overwhelming at times. Concerns about the size of your penis, your ability to get an erection, your ability to maintain an erection as well as your ability to ensure your partner's sexual pleasure can all lead to significant feelings of anxiety. If you are feeling uncomfortable sexually, it can be tempting to simply go online. It is important to remember that sexual pleasure and sexual activity is an interaction, a process between two people. It is not a competition or a win/lose situation.

Sexual activity can be best described as sexual play. Sexual play is something that adults do together. It is a fun, enjoyable and low-stress activity. Sexual play leads to increased intimacy and feelings of pleasure.

Can you make sexual pleasure the goal, rather than sexual performance?

Generally, people can get stuck in their sexual expectations. Expectations tend to interrupt pleasure.

- What happens if you let go of your sexual expectations?
- Would you feel better or worse about yourself?
- What are your concerns about your ability to satisfy a sexual partner?

My sexual expectations

I believe that I should provide my adult sexual partner with:

_____

_____

_____

_____

I worry that I cannot satisfy my adult sexual partner because:

_____

_____

_____

_____

I avoid partnered sexual activities because:

_____

_____

_____

_____

I prefer solo sexual activities because:

_____

_____

_____

_____

Many people struggle with fears about having sex with a new partner. Some people worry about satisfying their partner, while other people worry about their body or the size of their genitals. Believe it or not, penis size is not an important element of sexual satisfaction. Your ability to be content with your body and to engage in sexually satisfying activities that please you both is a more helpful focus. If you want to enhance your feeling of confidence in sexual situations, take the time to read some self-help books on the topic of sexuality. Try books identified in the Recommended Readings section of this workbook such as: *She Comes First* by Dr. Ian Kerner, *Sex for Dummies* by Dr. Ruth Westheimer or *The Man's Guide to Women* by Dr. John Gottman, Dr. Julie Schwartz Gottman and their colleagues. There are many good books that you can explore to help you feel more capable in your sexual activities with an adult partner. If you don't like to read, most of these books are available as audiobooks as well!

Sexual performance concerns are often related to your ability to get and maintain an erection. An erection is a reflex. It is not something that you simply command. Your body is not a machine, and erections will come and go during sexual activity. Some qualities of your erections will change with age, due to physical health concerns or due to medication use. If you are concerned about the quality of your erections, it is best to consult with a local sexual therapist for additional assistance. If you are certain that you do suffer from erectile dysfunction, a difficulty getting and maintaining erections, this is a problem that you can resolve. There are specific strategies to deal with this problem, including talking to your doctor to evaluate your physical health, talking to a counselor to address feelings of anxiety as well as talking specifically with a sexual therapist. A good book to read that addresses erectile dysfunction is called *Coping with Erectile Dysfunction* by Dr. Michael Metz and Dr. Barry McCarthy (2004). There are also medications that can help address erectile concerns.

You may have specific concerns related to sexual arousal, delayed ejaculation and/or ejaculating too fast. These problems can also be addressed. Delayed ejaculation means that you do not ejaculate or that it takes you a long time to ejaculate. Some men tend to ejaculate too fast, while others struggle to ejaculate. Enhancing your mindfulness during sex, focusing on your physical sensations and paying attention to the things that are sexually arousing to you is important. Explore your sexual concerns in more detail with a sexual therapist. You may also wish to speak to your physician and request a referral to see a urologist if it is recommended. A book that helps address premature ejaculation is written by Dr. Barry McCarthy and Dr. Michael Metz (2004). Seek an experienced sexual therapist for additional assistance with addressing your sexual performance concerns.

As we discuss sexual issues, we must also address sexual orientation and gender identity. Sexual orientation means the type of partner that you prefer: same-sex, opposite sex or a combination of both. Gender identity means your identification as male, female or another label that makes you most comfortable. Sometimes people struggle with their gender identity. This can lead to difficulties with sexual adjustment and functioning. In other cases, people struggle with their sexual orientation. For example, you know that you prefer same-sex partners; however, for many reasons, you don't want to admit that fact. You may also prefer both men and women but are ashamed to discuss the topic of bisexuality. In some cases, people who struggle with their gender identity and/or their sexual orientation pretend to be someone that they are not; they deny their true feelings. The problem is that it can then become tempting to spend time online rather than addressing these concerns.

Jerry is an adult male. He is straight; everyone knows that this is the case. Jerry has always dated girls. He makes sexual comments about girls and puts down gays in his community. Jerry grew up in a small town. It was not safe to be gay in his town. Everyone knew that being gay was not ok. As a teen, Jerry noticed that he had sexual thoughts about other guys. He ignored them. He pretended that he was not attracted to men. Eventually, he got married to the right girl, the girl everyone expected him to marry. Jerry turned to the Internet to masturbate. He would masturbate to pictures of men. He started watching more gay porn. His use of pornography expanded over time, and he started using increasingly different images. He began to use pictures of underage boys. He was eventually arrested by police for using CSEM.

Jerry knew he had sexual interests that were not in line with his lifestyle. He denied his sexuality and his sexual interests. He never talked about it. Once Jerry admitted that he was gay, he was able to create a life that better suited him. He moved to a larger city and developed friendships with people who didn't care whether he liked girls or guys. He was much happier and found it easy to avoid CSEM use. If you are like Jerry, it will be important to identify your true sexual interests. Are they legal? If so, would it be harmful to acknowledge your sexual interests rather than hiding them and only accessing them online? Is there a way to explore your sexual interests without harming yourself or others? Reach out for help to address this very important sexual issue.

My sexual interests include:

_____

_____

_____

_____

_____

My sexual problems are:

_____

_____

_____

_____

_____

I will address my sexual problems by:

_____

_____

_____

_____

_____

In the next chapter, we will discuss the impact of relationships on your life.

CHAPTER SUMMARY

- Learn the rules of sexual consent. Remember the importance of following legal expectations whether or not you agree with the legal definitions that are in place in your jurisdiction.
- Sexual interest in children does not go away. If you have this interest, identify the steps you need to take to manage your attraction.
- Sex is play. Make your sexual expectations reasonable and achievable.
- Carefully consider whether it is safe for you to use adult pornography.
- Sexual performance issues can be addressed. Seek help if you are struggling with specific concerns related to your sexual performance.
- Read or listen to self-help books if you want to increase your confidence about satisfying your sexual partner.
- Concerns about your sexual orientation or your gender identity can be very difficult. Reach out for help to discuss these issues in more detail.

REFERENCES

McCarthy, B. W., & Metz, M. E. (2004). *Coping with premature ejaculation: How to overcome PE, please your partner and have great sex.* Oakland, CA: New Harbinger Publications.

Metz, M. E., & McCarthy, B. W. (2004). *Coping with erectile dysfunction: How to regain confidence and enjoy great sex.* Oakland, CA: New Harbinger Publications.

NOTE

1 Holt, K., Kissinger, J., Spickler, C., & Roush, V. (2021). Pornography use and sexual offending: An examination of perceptions of role and risk. *International Journal of Offender Therapy and Comparative Criminology*, 1–25. https://doi.org/10.1177/0306624X211049183

9

Relationships, Community and Loneliness

CLINICIAN GUIDE

Relationships are the building blocks of our lives. Most of us yearn for social connection. Often clients have isolated themselves for many reasons, whether it is situational events (loss of family, toxic families or death), personal deficiencies (inadequate social skills, conflicts in relationships), poor relationship history (loss in relationships, unsuccessful relationships), relationship anxiety (social anxiety or a refusal to engage in intimate relationships) and/or any other elements. Understanding the importance of relationships, discussing difficulties in relationships, improving relationships and creating sustainable relationships are all part of the work in this chapter.

The first step is to define and understand what we mean by *relationships*. People can have very different understandings of what is meant by the term "relationship". Different types of relationships need to be identified and discussed with the client while also emphasizing how relationships tend to develop over time. Often our clients do not realize how frequently they misstep when navigating the developmental stages of relationships. The importance of understanding the social skills connected to interacting with strangers, familiar faces, acquaintances, casual friends, friends, best friends and partners needs to be outlined. This process allows clients to identify difficulties in their social behaviors. Often, people either move too fast through the stages of a relationship, or they do not increase the level of intimacy in their relationships. As such, in this chapter the clinician should start by reviewing the various types of relationships (e.g. strangers, a familiar face, an acquaintance, a casual friend, a friend, a best friend, a romantic partner) and how relationships may or may not develop and become more emotionally intimate over time. The definitions of these types of relationships are important to define clearly for the client. Please refer to the client workbook portion of this chapter for a full overview of these types of relationships and their corresponding definitions.

As the client reflects on the nature of their relationships and their understanding of the different types of relationships, they may begin to see gaps in their social connections. These gaps are identified by clients as they explore the nature of intimacy. The sad fact is that just because someone is an auntie, a mom or a wife does not necessarily guarantee that there is an intimate connection. The client may have people in their life but upon reflection, these people are not intimate, close or trustworthy. Helping the client create more intimacy in their lives is the first step to changing their relationship patterns.

DOI: 10.4324/9781003388142-10

Once relationships are well defined by the client, it is important to start identifying the nature of the relationships in their lives and how to increase both intimacy and trust in their personal interactions. Often, CSEM clients are very isolated. As a consequence of their social isolation, they begin to build online communities. As they do, they forsake creating close relationships in their community. While online relationships can be quite important and fulfilling, they do not preclude the need for offline relationships. Relying only on online communities can lead to more intense feelings of loneliness, inadequacy and boredom, which are risk-relevant treatment targets for CSEM users (Paquette, Chopin, & Fortin, 2022; Merdian et al., 2020). Openly discussing loneliness and creating a plan to combat feelings of loneliness is an important treatment target.

Addressing how to develop relationships and engage in social interactions is also an important part of this chapter. Does your client have good basic social skills? If not, where do they struggle: initiating relationships, maintaining relationships or ending toxic relationships? Being open with your client about their self-care, communication style and conversational skills is essential. Creating successful social experiences can enhance feelings of competence and resilience. If your client has sufficient social skills, encourage them to practice their skills by participating in local activities, joining community groups and/or community events.

We must consider personal, social and/or cultural expectations when exploring relationships with the client. Maintaining your awareness of various cultural and social expectations is important, as these may impact your client's relationship expectations. What is expected in relationships from the client's perspective? What are they looking for in a partner and how do they define healthy and unhealthy relationships? Knowing the cultural and community norms for your client is important when discussing relationships.

Everyone has a different relationship template. Ensure that your discussions with the client are focused on their relationship templates, rather than your own. Bring an open and non-judgmental approach to this conversation. Relationships can involve one partner or multiple partners. How do your beliefs as a clinician impact your openness to discussions about open relationships and/or monogamous relationships? What will work for the client? Focus on the elements that work best for the client, particularly when defining the concept of healthy relationships.

There are particular behaviors that predict relationship dissolution, such as showing contempt, criticism, defensiveness and emotional withdrawal (Gottman & Silver, 2015). These divorce predictors, as defined by Dr. Gottman and colleagues, are one way to explore unhealthy relationships from a research-based perspective. Building trust within relationships is another important issue when discussing relationships. Clinicians are referred to Dr. Gottman's work on the science of creating and rebuilding trust in relationships (see Gottman, 2011 and Gottman & Gottman, 2017 for details). A note about ADHD and relationships: there are unique relationship challenges that apply to people with ADHD. We refer you to literature specific to ADHD and relationships to assist these clients (see Orlov, 2010 for details).

In addition, the presence of toxic relationships, including domestic abuse as defined by physical, verbal or emotional abuse either as a victim or a perpetrator, needs to be explored with the client. These dynamics can occur regardless of gender. Investigate for the presence of domestic violence in the client's history. Chaotic, conflict-driven relationships, where obvious problems are not being addressed, can be very harmful. Identifying red flags in relationships, including controlling partners and/or partners who are unavailable to engage in truly intimate relationships, can be addressed as needed. Refer your client to domestic violence programs specifically designed for perpetrators or victims as needed.

Some clients frequently choose unavailable partners, or they become very anxious in relationships due to previous attachment injuries which can create problems in their current relationships. Discussing adult attachment style theory can enhance this work (see Cassidy & Shaver, 2016 and Hazan & Shaver, 1987 for details). We encourage you to find ways to discuss positive relationship choices using a research-based approach when you are exploring the topic of relationships.

Talk openly about dating, dating skills, and who they might want to date. Basic dating skills should be reviewed. Assist clients as needed to connect with helpful resources to address these concerns (see Ansari & Klinenberg, 2015 to explore these concepts). Clinicians also need to help the client clearly define what kind of relationship might be risky for them. For example, can they court a partner who has access to children? What type of partner would be a healthy choice for them? Assist the client to determine safe dating parameters.

Some clients would prefer to avoid rejection. Social anxiety can be a real impediment to establishing positive relationships. Be sure to examine whether this is true for your client. Should your client struggle significantly with social anxiety, seek additional mental health support.

Taking the time to explore relationship expectations and dynamics is an important treatment target. Relationships, loneliness, social anxiety, dating as well as establishing and maintaining positive relationships are essential topics to address as it relates to the ongoing use of CSEM. We encourage you to use additional resources related to relationship building. There are some suggestions in the recommended reading portion of this workbook, or you can rely on the relationship theory that best fits your clinical practice. Many CSEM clients require significant attention to their relationships and/or to the lack of relationships in their lives. We encourage you to work with the client to help them create satisfying and sustainable relationships in their lives.

REFERENCES

Ansari, A., & Klinenberg, E. (2015). *Modern romance*. New York: Penguin Press.

Cassidy, J., & Shaver, P. R. (2016). *Handbook of attachment: Theory, research and clinical application*. New York: Guilford Press.

Gottman, J. M. (2011). *The science of trust: Emotional attunement for couples*. New York: WW. Norton.

Gottman, J. M., & Gottman, J. (2017). The natural principles of love. *Journal of Family Theory and Review, 9*, 7–26. https://doi.org/10.1111/jftr.12182

Gottman, J. M., & Silver, N. (2015). *The seven principles for making marriage work*. New York: Harmony Press.

Hazan, C., & Shaver, P. (1987). Romantic love conceptualized as an attachment process. *Journal of Personality and Social Psychology, 52*, 511–524.

Merdian, H. L., Perkins, D. E., Dustagheer, E., & Glorney, E. (2020). Development of a case formulation model for individuals who have viewed, distributed, and/or shared child sexual exploitation material. *International Journal of Offender Therapy and Comparative Criminology, 64*(10–11), 1055–1073. https://doi.org/10.1177/0306624X17748067

Orlov, M. (2010). *The ADHD effect on marriage: Understand and rebuild your relationship in six steps*. Plantation, FL: Speciality Press/A.D.D. Warehouse.

Paquette, S., Chopin, J., & Fortin, F. (2022). Child sexual exploitation material offenders, one-size-fits-all for? Exploring tailored clinical dimensions based on cognitive and behavioural criminogenic factors. *Criminal Behaviour & Mental Health, 32*(2), 100–113. https://doi.org/10.1002/cbm.2242

CLIENT WORKBOOK

Learning Objectives

In this chapter, you will:

a) learn about various types of relationships
b) reflect on the level of intimacy in your relationships
c) learn about the importance of your online associates
d) learn how to reduce loneliness
e) identify red flags in relationships
f) create a plan to improve your relationships

Relationships are a very important part of life. As we will see in this chapter, relationships can have a big impact on your life. Maybe you currently have no relationships or perhaps only have a few. On the other hand, you may have many relationships; however, they may or may not be satisfying for you. In this chapter, we will explore the importance of relationships and strategies to improve the relationships in your life.

About Relationships

First, and most importantly, let's define what we are talking about. The word "relationships" can lead to confusion and misunderstanding. Are we talking about sexual partners, romantic partners, family members or what? Let's look at the different types of relationships!

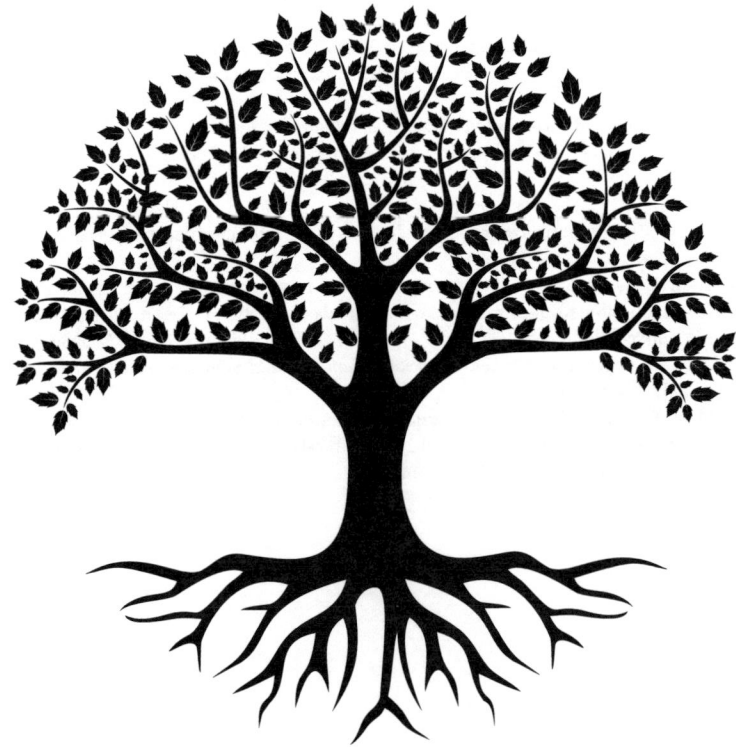

Figure 9.1 Our relationships change and grow over time

Here are the different types of relationships.

Strangers: A stranger is someone you don't know. You have no information about them. You typically don't share information with a stranger outside of making superficial enquiries (if you are a Canadian, you might ask "how are you?" without expecting an answer). You might talk about the weather or make a sports comment while waiting for your turn in a line.

Familiar face: A familiar face is someone that you have seen before, but you don't really know them. If you are in an urban setting, this might be the person behind the counter at the coffee shop. In a rural setting, it might be someone from the other village that you have seen, or you might know a member of their family. You typically don't share much information with a familiar face, except for making superficial small talk.

Acquaintance: An acquaintance is someone that you know, but not well. You might know a few things about them, but you do not know very much about their personal life. You typically do not share much personal information with an acquaintance, but you may share some general facts about your life.

Casual friend: A casual friend is someone you know a bit better. You will know more things about their life. You may go out with them as part of a group or get together with them on occasion. A casual friend begins to take some space in your life, and you begin to share more information with them about you.

Friend: A friend is someone that you know well. You will share personal information with them, and they will share personal information with you. You begin to feel emotionally close to them and may depend on them for emotional or perhaps even support with concrete needs like a place to live, financial help or help moving.

Best friend: A best friend is someone that you know extremely well, and they know you extremely well. You share personal information with a best friend. They know about the good and the bad aspects of your life. You are open with them, feel comfortable with them, share with them and depend on them as an integral part of your life.

Partner: A partner is a person with whom you have chosen to share your life. This person knows you in depth and you know them in depth as well. You are close to them and talk about vulnerable topics. They know all aspects of your life.

We start all our relationships as strangers, and we get to know people over time. As we gain trust and intimacy within our relationships, we begin to share more personal information with each other. The level of intimacy in a relationship can improve, it can stay the same or it can deteriorate. We often do not consider how our relationships change and grow over time.

Have you ever had an experience where someone has "overshared" in a public place or during an initial meeting? How did it feel? Sometimes, it feels odd when we communicate with someone in a way that ignores the stage we are at in the relationship. There are community, cultural and social norms that impact the way we engage with each other. You may find that the stages outlined here may serve you as general guidelines rather than firm rules, depending on your cultural and community expectations.

Consider Your Relationships

When you look at your various relationships, you may notice that you have a good group of close people in your life, or you may notice that you tend to get stuck at a particular stage of relationship with people. Perhaps you have developed a long-term live-in relationship, but you and your partner have not truly progressed to a deeper level of intimacy. Let's consider your relationships.

George was considering his relationships based on the list here. He has always thought that he had many friends. George has many people he talks to at work and at his local hangout. He is considered to be very friendly and chatty. George noticed that most of his interactions were at the acquaintance level. He tended not to share very much personal information with people, keeping things superficial. He remembered that when he was in the hospital, there was no one that he was comfortable calling for help. He began to think that he might want to tell people more about himself and ask them more about their personal lives the next time he went out.

It is important to notice what kind of relationships you have.

- Do you have very few or no relationships?
- Do you mainly interact with strangers and familiar faces?
- Do you have many superficial relationships, such as acquaintances, but no close friends?
- How do you grow your relationships: very slowly or do you move too fast?

An important note: just because someone is an aunt, uncle, mother, father, brother, sister, partner, coworker or family member does not guarantee that they have attained a level of intimacy in their relationship with you. A social title does not mean that they have an honored place in your life. In other words, you may have a coworker with whom you have developed a close friendship, while you have another coworker who remains a familiar face. Or you may have a wife who is essentially a casual friend because you don't talk and don't share personal information with each other. Family members are typically expected to be in positions of high intimacy; however, this is not always the case. For example, you may have poor relationships with parents or siblings. Despite the label of "family", you might not have a close or an intimate relationship with your family members. It is important to focus on the level of intimacy in the relationship rather than the label. This will be important as you reflect on the relationships in your life.

What Level of Intimacy Have You Developed With the People in Your Life?

List your relationships and the degree of intimacy that is present. Use the definitions listed here. Explain why you think you have reached that degree of intimacy with this person.

0 = Stranger or Familiar Face definition – no intimacy
5 = Casual friend definition – partial intimacy
10 = Best friend definition and/or partner definition – full intimacy

Relationship 1
Name_____
Level of intimacy 0 . . . 1 . . . 2 . . . 3 . . . 4 . . . 5 . . . 6 . . . 7 . . . 8 . . . 9 . . . 10

_____

_____

_____

Relationship 2
Name_____
Level of intimacy 0 . . . 1 . . . 2 . . . 3 . . . 4 . . . 5 . . . 6 . . . 7 . . . 8 . . . 9 . . . 10

_____

_____

_____

Relationship 3
Name_____
Level of intimacy 0 . . . 1 . . . 2 . . . 3 . . . 4 . . . 5 . . . 6 . . . 7 . . . 8 . . . 9 . . . 10

_____

_____

_____

Relationship 4
Name_____
Level of intimacy 0 . . . 1 . . . 2 . . . 3 . . . 4 . . . 5 . . . 6 . . . 7 . . . 8 . . . 9 . . . 10

_____

_____

_____

Relationship 5
Name_____
Level of intimacy 0 . . . 1 . . . 2 . . . 3 . . . 4 . . . 5 . . . 6 . . . 7 . . . 8 . . . 9 . . . 10

_____

_____

_____

Relationship 6
Name_____
Level of intimacy 0 . . . 1 . . . 2 . . . 3 . . . 4 . . . 5 . . . 6 . . . 7 . . . 8 . . . 9 . . . 10

_____

_____

_____

Relationship 7
Name_____
Level of intimacy 0 . . . 1 . . . 2 . . . 3 . . . 4 . . . 5 . . . 6 . . . 7 . . . 8 . . . 9 . . . 10

_____

_____

_____

Relationship 8
Name_____
Level of intimacy 0 . . . 1 . . . 2 . . . 3 . . . 4 . . . 5 . . . 6 . . . 7 . . . 8 . . . 9 . . . 10

_____

_____

_____

When you review your list, what do you notice? What type of relationships do you typically have? Where do you struggle in your relationships? How can you improve the level of intimacy in your relationships? We will examine some common relationship difficulties for people who use CSEM before creating a plan to improve your relationships.

Often people who have accessed CSEM have maintained online relationships that have encouraged offending behaviors. This includes online relationships with other people who use CSEM, other people who share or post CSEM, other people who make comments that encourage the sexualization of children as well as other people who normalize or encourage online sexual behaviors. Online relationships are difficult on many levels. The first and most obvious concern is actually knowing who you are communicating with. People can lie about their personal circumstances, gender, age and other various aspects of their personal history and current lifestyle. This can be much harder to detect when you are only communicating online. Online relationships that involve face-to-face communications can help increase the level of personal knowledge that you have about someone, but it can still be difficult to truly get to know them and their lifestyle. Most importantly, people will say and do things online that they would not do in their community.

My Online Associates

It is now time to consider the nature of the online interactions you were having when you were searching for CSEM. We are assuming that you no longer have any communication with the people you were accessing CSEM with in the past; however, if this is not the case, reflect on these ongoing relationships. What types of people were you interacting with?

Who were your online associates?

_____

_____

What level of intimacy did you believe you had with your online associates?

_____

_____

What types of activities did you engage in with your online associates?

_____

_____

Were your online associates making positive choices or harmful choices for themselves and/or others?

_____

_____

Were your online associates actively encouraging you to view CSEM?

_____

_____

Were your online associates supportive of the sexualization of children?

_____

_____

Do you have online associates that you hope to continue to communicate with in the future?

_____

_____

The people you are communicating with online, the people on the other side of the computer screen, are real people! Just like the victims in the images are REAL children. When you forget that things online are real, you can make poor choices. Just as you would not hang around people in your community who were negative influences in your life, being with negative people online is a problem. Would you typically socialize with criminals in the community? Do you think that it is ok to abuse children? Do you think that it is ok to break the law? If you do not, why would you associate with people who are making negative choices online?

When you examine your relationships, you may notice that all of your relationships were with online acquaintances. If all of your relationships occur online, it is time to reach out to people in your local community. Fear and anxiety can keep you from establishing relationships with others in your community. If you are struggling to find friends in your community, it is important that you address this problem.

As you explore your relationships, you may also notice that you are more comfortable interacting with children than adults. Sometimes children can seem safer than adults. Children are more easily impressed, they can be less judgmental, they ask fewer questions and they may show affection more easily. You may prefer to socialize with younger children, young teens or older teens. This is risky.

Paul is a 40-year-old man. He enjoys skateboarding and going to the movies. Paul is often frustrated with people his own age. They never want to do anything fun. They are always so serious. Paul doesn't feel like he fits in, so he seeks out youths instead. Youths don't ask so many questions and they are impressed with the fact that he can buy alcohol and that he has his own place. They don't criticize him for wanting to do youthful activities or making bad jokes. As a result, Paul spends most of his time with younger people.

If this seems familiar to you, what is occurring in your relationships with people your own age? Sometimes childhood bullying or childhood abuse can contribute to a fear of rejection and interfere with a person's readiness and ability to establish peer relationships. Other times, feelings of failure or feeling a lack of accomplishment can lead to avoiding other adults. It is important to notice your tendency to approach children or teens for relationships rather than adults. If you notice this, we encourage you to examine the issues that have interfered in the development of peer-age relationships. The goal is to develop age-appropriate relationships. It will be important not to approach children or youths in the community or online, but to find adult partners with whom you can share healthy activities. There are other adults who will enjoy the same activities, although you may have to work a bit harder to find them. Establishing positive relationships with adults will be a critical step toward change.

Loneliness

Many people struggle with loneliness. People live more independently, there is less pressure to marry and many people are living on their own, outside of extended family environments. Loneliness is real.[1] How often do you feel lonely?

> Tom has had a happy life. He can't understand how he has gotten himself in trouble for viewing CSEM. This is not who he is. Tom lives alone. He is a widower. He was married for many years. His wife's death was hard for him. He tried to connect with their usual friends after her death, but it was too hard. He was the lone man out and it reminded him of his loss. He was alone. Tom began to spend lots of time online. He filled his time surfing, chatting and masturbating online. This eventually led to the police being at his door to arrest him. He recognizes his grief but has difficulty acknowledging how profoundly lonely he was feeling after his wife's death. It was very difficult having to adjust to living alone.

Loneliness hits us hard for many different reasons. Maybe, like Tom, you have lost a partner, maybe you have never established a romantic relationship or maybe you are married but feel lonely because the intimacy in your relationship has faded away over the years.

Combating loneliness is an important step as it will help you change your computer habits and your viewing of CSEM. Remember Charles from Chapter 5? He noticed that he was masturbating first thing in the morning. To change his habits, he joined a local running group. It got him out of the house, and those new social connections were essential in improving his mood and his decision-making. We all need some amount of social connection. We all need to be busy doing things that give us purpose.

What can you do to reduce your feelings of loneliness? Go out and meet new people, try new activities, let people get to know you and be vulnerable enough to build relationships with others. While this can be scary, it pays off when you are no longer feeling lonely within your life. If one of your longstanding vulnerabilities involves a sexual attraction to children, focus on finding new relationships with people who do not have children in their lives.

Let's start with identifying things that you like to do. For now, do not to focus on the barriers to trying different activities (e.g., I will be uncomfortable, I don't dance, I can't afford it, etc.). Focus on the things that you might enjoy, and from there you can find alternatives that would suit your personal lifestyle.

Examples of activities

- Car shows
- CrossFit training
- Sports teams
- Gym membership or group exercise classes

- Local activity centers
- Gaming groups
- Magic: The Gathering card game
- Dungeons and Dragons groups
- Board game groups
- Bowling
- Coffee shops
- Group videogame sessions
- Organized sports
- Book clubs
- Scrapbooking clubs
- Chess clubs
- Poker clubs or card game groups
- Horse, dog, and/or other animal groups (e.g., equestrian activities, fly ball clubs for dogs)
- Dance classes (line dancing, ballroom dancing, salsa dancing, etc.)
- Hiking clubs
- Reenactment groups (Middle Ages, military, or history-based events)
- Ski or snowboarding groups
- Running groups
- Musical activities (musicians, choirs, volunteer at music festivals)
- Learning a new instrument or developing a musical interest
- Volunteering in the community
- Inviting people to your home or to a local restaurant for a meal
- Create weekly suppers and invite guests (set time and rotate the menu)
- Cooking classes
- Mindfulness groups
- Spiritual groups, church services or faith-based activities
- Take a class or pursue a new educational activity
- Go for a drive with the goal of finding new local activities or events
- Visit an art gallery
- Go to a show, concert or movies where you might interact with someone new
- Astronomy groups
- Darts group or billiards group
- Bingo groups
- Other: _____
- Other: _____
- Other: _____

What activities come to mind as possible things to do in your community?

_____

_____

_____

_____

In many communities, you can find gatherings by looking online. Visit www.meetup.com to access free or very inexpensive gatherings in your area. You can also search for "things to do in my area" to find new ideas for local activities.

Now that you have thought about some alternatives, make a list. Notice that you don't have to be sure you'll love any activity yet! Just be willing to try something new. A new activity might lead you down the path to finding other activities that you had not considered, activities that are truly enjoyable for you.

Here are some hobbies or activities that I am willing to try:

_____

_____

_____

_____

_____

A great way to combat loneliness is to get a pet. Animals bring us motivation to get up; they are a living being that needs you and offers lots of affection and purpose. Animals are a wonderful way to connect to the community too as there are many animal-focused activities (e.g., your local dog park, pet-focused community groups and activities), as well as positive daily habits such as walking your pet, socializing with your pet and caring for your pet. If you are not able to have a pet in your home, consider volunteering at a pet center (e.g. community pet shows, animal rescue centers, animal therapy clinics or veterinary clinics in your area), or you can offer pet walking and/or pet sitting services to local pet owners. If you are not ready to add a new person to your life, perhaps it is time to add a pet to your life!

As we discussed earlier in this chapter, it may be that you hesitate to try new activities because you are uncomfortable meeting new people. Social anxiety is real. It can feel bad to be in new social environments. Letting the anxiety win, however, does nothing to help you in the long run. It is important to review the information on emotions management in Chapter 6 if this is a problem for you.

> Tim is a very shy person. He has always been shy. His family has stories about how shy he was as a child. Talking to people is just hard. He gets much better once he has gotten to know someone. He has a job that requires him to talk to others on his team and he can do that. He avoids situations where he has to talk to new people. As a result, Tim has not dated at all. He does not know what he would say on a first date. Tim would like to have a partner in his life, but he is fearful of trying to date.

Dating

Dating can be hard. Just like maintaining a relationship with a long-term partner, we all need to put some time and energy aside to create, build and maintain our relationships. Exploring dating strategies is outside the scope of this workbook, but there are some good resources that can help you.

Remember that dating is a way to get to know someone. What are they like? Do you feel comfortable in their presence? Are they interested in getting to know you? Online dating can be particularly challenging. It is time-consuming and requires some effort (for example, taking the time to create your profile, reading through other people's profiles as well as having the ability to meet new people at a local coffee shop or restaurant on a regular basis). If you are going to explore online dating, it is important that you build a reasonable profile with pictures that show you in a positive light. Be willing to explore different dating sites and focus on trying to meet someone in your community. There are tips on how to navigate the online dating world in the book *Modern Romance* by Aziz Ansari and Eric Klinenberg (2015), as well as other resources in the Recommended Readings section of this workbook.

Alternatively, the more activities that you engage in outside the home, the better. Think about all those leisure activities you listed to combat feelings of loneliness! They can also help you meet new people with whom you might want to spend more time. In most communities, there are many singles activities, singles travel groups, singles associations and singles meet-ups that you can join. Get out there and try! This is a great way to deal with the anxiety of dating, and it can help you achieve your relationship goals. Remember, there is someone out there who will enjoy meeting you; the trick is not to give up and to keep trying!

Basic relationship skills involve good hygiene, paying attention to your physical health and addressing your mental health. How do you look and feel today? Is your body sluggish and/or not at its best? It might be time to take care of your physical health. Checking in with your physician, seeing a dentist, and/or adding some new items to your wardrobe may be timely as you explore the possibility of new relationships. Talk with your therapist, your friends and/or your family about how you present yourself. Is there anything that you could improve to help you feel better about dating and finding a partner?

Let's consider some questions to help you navigate the land of dating.

What do I need to do in order to get myself prepared to date?

_____

_____

_____

What type of lifestyle or type of relationship do I want with a partner?

_____

_____

_____

_____

Describe a typical day if I was with the right partner for me:

_____

_____

_____

_____

What qualities do I have that would make me a great partner?

_____

_____

_____

_____

What are things that I cannot accept in my future relationships?

_____

_____

_____

What has hindered my past relationships?

_____

_____

_____

_____

What can I change to improve my future relationships?

_____

_____

_____

_____

Initiating a relationship is the first step. The second step is to ensure that the relationships in our lives work well for us. How do you know what a good relationship is for you? Everyone's criteria are different. A relationship that works well for one person might not necessarily work well for another person. Throughout this section we will focus on romantic relationships. If you do not wish to pursue romantic relationships, the information here may still be relevant to you. Simply focus on applying the material to the type of relationship you are seeking to establish or to maintain in your life.

What do you want in your romantic relationships? How do you determine what a good relationship or a bad relationship is for you? Often when a relationship ends, we realize that there were indicators that it was not a good fit.

Common Red Flags in Relationships:

- Your friends and/or family members are telling you that there is a problem in the relationship, or they have a concern about your relationship
- You do not feel safe sharing your thoughts or feelings with your partner
- You are unhappy in the relationship
- You do not feel heard in the relationship
- Your needs are not met within the relationship
- There is physical, emotional, financial and/or sexual abuse in the relationship
- There is illegal activity occurring within the relationship
- There are problems with substance abuse
- There is infidelity in the relationship
- There is an active, untreated mental health condition within the relationship

Let's explore a few common problems that can occur in relationships.

At times, people avoid obvious problems in their lives. If this becomes their main way of addressing difficulties, we refer to this as *coping by avoidance*. People who avoid make it very difficult to fix problems in relationships. They won't identify whether they are unhappy or unsatisfied in the relationship, they won't be willing to address problems and they won't inform their partners if they are thinking about ending the relationship. It becomes very difficult to build relationships with partners who are avoidant. Does this seem familiar to you? Has this been a pattern for you or in your partners? If so, it will be important to discuss this pattern with your treatment provider and/or a couples counselor.

Sometimes people struggle with setting boundaries and/or clearly stating their needs in relationships. This can lead to people either being too passive or being too aggressive in their relationships. If you struggle with being passive in your relationships, it means that you don't tend to tell your partner what you think, feel, need or want from them. It is important to find ways to openly communicate your thoughts, opinions and concerns. In contrast, if you struggle with being overly aggressive in your relationships, this means that you communicate from a position of power, trying to exert control over your partner. This will lead to your partner feeling unsafe and more likely to not openly address any relationship concerns as they occur. Alternatively, it may lead to a relationship that has lots of conflict and animosity. There are resources in the Recommended Readings part of this workbook to improve your communication style in relationships, including identifying and setting boundaries, as well as books on anger management. If domestic violence has been a part of your past or your current relationships, it will be important to address this issue clearly with your treatment provider.

How have you contributed to reduced intimacy in your past relationships? Some problems that can create barriers to intimacy include a lack of self-esteem, a reluctance to share personal information, a passive communication style that undermines the ability to work through problems in relationships, problems with anger and/or aggression that result in others being scared and not wanting to get emotionally close to you, a history of lying or deceit that results in a lack of trust and alcohol or drug problems that have led to a lack of dependability. In addition, breaches of trust also occur as a result of your use of CSEM.

Repairing trust in relationships takes time and energy. Acknowledge your behaviors and seek to repair relationships if others are willing to reconnect with you; we will discuss this further in Chapter 12. If you have a history of infidelity in relationships, you will need to identify ways to appropriately apologize for your behaviors. The book *Get Out of the Doghouse* by Robert Weiss (2017) may help you explore how to apologize and address your past choices. In addition, finding community resources to assist you in navigating these concerns is recommended. Addressing your relationship concerns will be a powerful tool to help improve your life.

Let's examine the role of difficulties in your relationships. What barriers to intimacy have you faced in the past? What barriers to intimacy do you currently face?

Which of the following have been barriers to intimacy in your relationships?

. . . .
1   2   3   4   5

1 = Untrue of me
2 = Sometimes true of me
3 = Often true of me
4 = True of me
5 = Very true of me

1) Difficulties with trust	1	2	3	4	5
2) Difficulties with jealousy	1	2	3	4	5
3) Not speaking up about my thoughts and feelings	1	2	3	4	5
4) Not asking about the thoughts and feelings of others	1	2	3	4	5
5) Focusing on what I want and not paying enough attention to what others would like or need	1	2	3	4	5
6) Lying and keeping secrets	1	2	3	4	5
7) Using drugs and alcohol	1	2	3	4	5
8) Using anger and violence in my relationships	1	2	3	4	5
9) Other:	1	2	3	4	5
10) Other:	1	2	3	4	5

What were the red flags in your past relationships?

_____

_____

_____

What red flags to you see in your current relationship?

_____

_____

_____

What other difficulties can you identify in your past and present relationships?

_____

_____

_____

_____

_____

_____

_____

It is important to note that arguments are not necessarily a symptom that there is a problem in your relationship. It is the ability to fix the relationship, to repair the relationship after an argument, that matters. You may enjoy reading *The Seven Principles for Making Marriage*

Work by Dr. John Gottman and Nan Silver (2015) for details about divorce predictors and the importance of repair within relationships.

Let's explore your relationships and your CSEM use. Here are some important themes to consider.

1) What needs were not met within my relationship before I started viewing CSEM?
2) What needs were not met within my relationship during the time I was viewing CSEM?
3) What relationship stress occurred in my relationship?
4) How did I deal with my anger within my relationships?
5) Did I start viewing CSEM before the relationship started or during the relationship?
6) Why did I not share my online difficulties with my partner? Why did I not ask for help?
7) Do I want to maintain my relationship?
8) What are the pros and cons of maintaining this relationship?
9) Is this relationship healthy for me?
10) If I want to maintain this relationship, how will I rebuild trust within my relationship moving forward, both for myself and for my partner?

People can use online activity and/or view CSEM as a way to avoid problems in their relationships. Sometimes it is a way to deal with feelings of anger toward your partner. These feelings of anger may not be something that you want to talk about. Being passive-aggressive means that when you are upset about something, you do something else to get back at the person. You hurt the person indirectly rather than talking openly about why you are upset. This is a dangerous habit because problems don't get resolved.

> Jerome was in a relationship for 4 years. He did not really like his partner. He felt that he "should" be in the relationship, but he didn't want to be there. He did not feel that his partner was very kind to him. Jerome never said anything when he was upset about something that his partner told him. Jerome would just stay quiet. He didn't want to have a fight. He never seemed to win fights. Jerome would go and spend time online when he was angry with his spouse. He would view CSEM and masturbate to feel better.

Does this scenario sound familiar to you? Managing your emotions and identifying your use of sex to cope with negative emotions is outlined in Chapter 6. It is very important to fix problems that are not working in your relationships. It might also be time to make an appointment to see your local couples counselor. If you would rather not attend couples counseling, you may enjoy going to relationship workshops. If ADHD is part of your relationship dynamic, there are specific programs and information that addresses this problem in more detail. Ask your treatment provider for local resources available to you.

Let's apply this information to your own circumstances:

1) What needs were not met within my relationship before I started viewing CSEM?

_____

_____

_____

_____

_____

_____

_____

2) What needs were not met within my relationship during the time I was viewing CSEM?

_____

_____

_____

_____

_____

_____

3) What relationship stress occurred during my relationship?

_____

_____

_____

_____

_____

_____

_____

4) How did I deal with my anger within my relationships?

_____

_____

_____

_____

5) Did I start viewing CSEM before the relationship started or during the relationship?

_____

_____

_____

_____

_____

_____

_____

6) Why did I not share my online difficulties with my partner? Why did I not ask for help?

_____

_____

_____

_____

_____

_____

_____

7) Do I want to maintain my relationship?

_____

_____

_____

_____

_____

_____

_____

8) What are the pros and cons of maintaining this relationship?

_____

_____

_____

_____

_____

_____

_____

9) Is this relationship healthy for me?

_____

_____

_____

_____

_____

_____

10) If I want to maintain this relationship, how will I rebuild trust within my relationship moving forward, both for myself and for my partner?

_____

_____

_____

_____

_____

_____

_____

It is time to create a plan to improve the quality and quantity of relationships in your life. Striving for increased intimacy in your relationships is a positive goal. Improving your satisfaction with the relationships in your life is also an important goal. Improving your relationships is one way to help you curb your use of CSEM. Be specific about your plan.

My plan to improve the relationships and the relationship intimacy in my life is:

_____

_____

_____

_____

_____

_____

_____

_____

_____

_____

_____

_____

_____

_____

_____

Improving your relationships is like any other skill. It helps to set goals for your relationships so that you know where you are trying to go and what you are trying to improve. Clearly identify your relationship goals.

I will set goals to track my improvements in my relationships. These goals will allow me to know if I am addressing the relationship problems in my life. My goals are:

1. _____

_____

_____

_____

2. _____

_____

_____

_____

3. _____

_____

_____

_____

4. _____

_____

_____

_____

5. _____

_____

_____

_____

6. _____

_____

_____

_____

Next, we will explore other roadblocks that might be getting in your way.

CHAPTER SUMMARY

- Relationships are important!
- Establish positive relationships with positive people.
- Build strong relationships that are consistent with the relationship stages listed in this chapter: stranger, familiar face, acquaintance, casual friend, friend, best friend and partner. Don't skip steps!
- Just as you would avoid negative people in the community, you must also avoid negative people online.
- If you prefer socializing with younger people, stop and start building relationships with adults instead.
- Ensure that you are happy in your relationships. Fix obvious problems in your relationships.
- If you are going to be dating, address basics such as your hygiene, your physical health, your mental health and consider the image that you are portraying to others.
- Identify how you have undermined the intimacy in your past and current relationships.
- Identify the relationship triggers that relate to your CSEM use. How will you address these relationship triggers moving forward?
- Set relationship goals to ensure that you are on track to improve your relationships.

REFERENCES

Ansari, A., & Klinenberg, E. (2015). *Modern romance*. New York: Penguin Press.
Gottman, J. M., & Silver, N. (2015). *The seven principles for making marriage work*. New York: Harmony Press.
Weiss, R. (2017). *Out of the doghouse: A step-by-step relationship-saving guide for men caught cheating*. Deerfield Beach, FL: Health Communications, Inc.

NOTE

1　Barreto, M., Victor, C., Hammond, C., Eccles, A., Richins, M. T., & Qualter, P. (2021). Loneliness around the world: Age, gender, and cultural differences in loneliness. *Personality and Individual Differences*, *169*, 110066, 2–6. https://doi.org/10.1016/j.paid.2020.110066.

10

Other Roadblocks

CLINICIAN GUIDE

As we identify other roadblocks on the client's treatment journey, it is useful to note that much of your treatment plan has now been accomplished. Taking the time to congratulate the client for work well done is a good way to begin this chapter. You may want to start with a summary of the work accomplished so far. Discuss how the client can reward themselves for changes made and motivation maintained throughout this process. If the client is lagging in their motivation, it may be time to focus on the gains made prior to adding new treatment objectives. It can also be useful to take a session or two to reflect on progress and to reward goals achieved. There is much to be proud of. As the client summarizes their gains, help them look for any elements that require continued attention.

In this chapter, we outline examples of common issues that may be relevant to the client (for example, problem-solving, sleep difficulties and childhood sexual abuse). Use the materials to discuss the sections that apply to the client. Whether the client is identifying these issues or different issues as outstanding to their treatment goals, develop a plan specific to the outstanding treatment targets. If their additional roadblocks are not in your area of expertise, refer the client to another practitioner to address these issues.

Sleep difficulties can be important to discuss with clients. In our clinical observations, we note that many clients used CSEM late at night and present with disrupted sleep cycles. Take the time to address any needs surrounding structure, routine and establishing healthy sleep habits. Ensure that common sleep problems such as sleep apnea, insomnia and/or any other sleep disorders are excluded as part of the client's difficulties. As with other issues discussed in this workbook, clients with ADHD often present with sleep difficulties and may have unique needs in this area (Aizenstros et al., 2019; Bijlenga, 2019). There are additional resources to assist with sleep concerns in the Recommended Readings section of this workbook.

Problem-solving strategies are useful to review with most clients involved in illegal behaviors. These strategies aim at improving the client's ability to identify problems accurately, create a plan to address these problems as well as implement a plan that will be effective to improve the problem in question. Clients who use CSEM may be particularly adept at using various forms of avoidance to escape problems rather than resolve them. Clients are encouraged to start exploring their use of avoidance and working on more productive ways to address their concerns. To achieve this goal, discussing boundaries and improving overall communication skills are two treatment targets to address when discussing problem-solving.

DOI: 10.4324/9781003388142-11

Assertiveness training and boundary setting may assist your client to move away from passively escaping life's problems. Discussing problem-solving skills with your client is encouraged in this section of treatment.

A note about working with childhood sexual abuse: this is trauma work. Ensure that the client is ready to work with this material before introducing it. Addressing childhood trauma is its own treatment protocol and can be quite difficult for most clients. It is likely that attempting to do this work, on top of the CSEM treatment plan, will be too much for many clients. This is completely normal. Doing trauma work specific to their childhood sexual abuse can wait until they are well situated in the maintenance phase of their CSEM treatment. If your client is not ready at that time, simply finish your CSEM treatment plan with a recommendation that the client start trauma counseling when they are ready to do so in the future. If trauma therapy is not your area of expertise, find an alternative practitioner who specializes in this area.

When discussing childhood sexual abuse and the relationship with CSEM use, we can only conclude that it is complicated. Clients have multiple reasons and explanations for their CSEM use and these can seem particularly complicated when it is related to their own past childhood victimization. Validating client concerns related to their past sexual victimization is an important therapeutic goal. We recommend avoiding getting into a debate about how their childhood victimization is connected to their present CSEM use. It can be more effective to focus on the ongoing victimization of other children by their use of CSEM, help them build empathy for the other victims, acknowledge the confusing arousal patterns that may develop as a result of their past experiences and explore the thinking errors that developed as a result of being groomed by offenders when they were children and youths. This approach avoids invalidating the client while preserving their motivation to change, dismantling any ongoing thinking errors related to their own victimization and moving them toward changing their illegal behaviors.

Addressing childhood sexual trauma requires specialized knowledge and needs to be carefully integrated into the treatment plan. It is best done when the client has the time and space to engage in trauma focused therapy.

During this stage of the treatment, the clinician is encouraged to reinforce the progress the client has made. Take time to identify any other elements that need to be addressed for the client to achieve their good life. The next few chapters will help the client summarize and finish their work.

REFERENCES

Aizenstros, J., Chan, E. S., Aizenstros, A., & May, T. (2019). Sleep in adults with ADHD – etiology, impact, and treatments. In H. Hiscock & E. Sciberras (Eds.), *Sleep and ADHD: An evidence based guide to assessment and treatment*. San Diego, CA: Academic Press. https://doi.org/10.1016/B978-0-12-814180-9.00012-0

Bijlenga, D., Vollebregt, M. A., Kooij, J. J. S., & Arns, M. (2019). The role of the circadian system in the etiology and pathophysiology of ADHD: Time to redefine ADHD? *ADHD Attention Deficit Hyperactivity Disorder, 11*, 5–19. https://doi.org/10.1007/s12402-018-0271-z

CLIENT WORKBOOK

Learning Objectives

In this chapter, you will:

a) learn the importance of sleep and how to improve it
b) learn the importance of problem-solving
c) reflect on the impact of childhood sexual abuse

There are other factors to consider in your journey toward making positive sexual choices and avoiding CSEM use in your life. In this chapter, we will discuss your sleep hygiene, general problem-solving skills and what to do if you have a history of childhood sexual abuse. If you identify other roadblocks that you wish to discuss, bring these to the attention of your treatment provider.

Sleep

Let's start with sleep.

Those who use CSEM frequently do so at night. You may have used CSEM while others were sleeping or as a way to cope with a lonely evening. You may also have used CSEM as a reward on weekends or after a long and tiring workday. Using a computer in the evening and/or at night can disrupt your sleep cycle.[1] When your sleep cycle is off, you tend to feel tired and it can be difficult to make good decisions. Sleep is important!

It might be time to reset your sleep cycle. Make sleep a priority in your life! Start going to sleep earlier. Allow your body to recharge and get the sleep you need to feel refreshed. If you are not waking refreshed, you may be struggling with sleep issues and/or health problems that are getting in your way.

Your lifestyle will impact your sleep. Alcohol and stimulant use (caffeine, drugs, food choices) can interrupt your sleep. While it is easy to believe that drinking alcohol is a helpful way to fall asleep, the use of alcohol before bed tends to disrupt your ability to stay asleep.[2] Stimulants will also disrupt your ability to get to sleep and stay asleep.[3]

Improve your sleep!

1. Practice gratitude at the end of each day. What am I thankful for today? Acknowledging small things can help you feel better and more at ease before bed.
2. Set and keep a regular sleep schedule. Develop a routine before going to sleep. Routines can remind you and your body that it is time for sleep. This can be tricky when you are a shift worker. When you are working hours that interfere with setting a regular sleep schedule, seek out additional assistance from a sleep expert. There is information specific to shift workers and many online blogs that also offer sleep strategies for shift workers.
3. Avoid electronic devices two to three hours before bed. The light emitted by computer screens, cellular phones and television has been found to stimulate the brain – exactly what you do not want to be doing before bed[4]! Create time without electronic stimulation. Ensure plenty of downtime to allow your body and mind to calm down before sleep.
4. Don't focus on anxiety-producing thoughts, scary thoughts, fearful thoughts or unhelpful thoughts prior to your bedtime. Thinking about how you will solve a particular problem may also create anxiety before bed. Some people imagine placing their

worries in a box and then placing that box on a shelf so that the box can be examined at a later time. Perhaps you might want to keep a notebook beside your bed to write down any problems or solutions that come to your mind before bed. This way, you can review and explore them in more detail the next morning when you are feeling rested and refreshed.

5. Getting proper aerobic exercise during the day can help you manage your mood and better manage your sleep patterns.

6. Holding a positive philosophy about your life, your goals and your personal purpose may also help improve your sleep. It may encourage you to remember the importance of following your sleep schedule. Are you happy about getting to the next day? Are you future-focused? Do you typically feel sad about having lost yet another day? Finding ways to stay focused and satisfied about your present and your future may also be helpful.

7. Keeping your room cool and dark may also assist you with falling asleep.

8. Remember that you cannot control when you fall asleep. This is a process that your body simply knows how to do. Allow the process to happen without trying to judge it, control it or force it. Getting upset about not falling asleep simply makes it harder to fall asleep.

9. Consider practicing meditation or deep breathing before bed to help your body and your mind calm down.

10. If there is evidence that you suffer from a sleep disorder such as sleep apnea, you should contact your physician for a proper assessment and treatment recommendations.

On a scale of 1–10, with one (1) being terrible sleep and ten (10) being awesome sleep, my sleep is generally:

1   2   3   4   5   6   7   8   9   10

As you start applying these skills, what do you notice? Are you identifying ongoing sleep issues? Here are some helpful questions to consider if you require additional assistance to resolve your sleep difficulties. Do you snore? Are you having difficulty falling asleep or staying asleep? Are you often tired during the day? Do you wake up feeling tired? If so, it may be time to consult a sleep expert. You may also enjoy the book *No More Sleepless Nights* by Dr. Peter Hauri & Dr. Shirley Linde. If you are concerned about the quality of your sleep, if you believe that you may have a sleep disorder or if you continue to struggle with your sleep hygiene, consult a sleep consultant for further assistance.

As discussed earlier, you may have been staying up late in order to avoid detection while using CSEM. If you have used your sleep time to engage in secretive behaviors or behaviors that you would rather hide from your partner and/or family, it is time to find ways to stay accountable during the night.

Do I need to use the Internet in the evenings? Yes_____/No _____
Do I need to use the Internet at night? Yes _____/No _____
How will I ensure that I will be held accountable for my Internet use in the evenings and/or during the night?

_____

_____

_____

Having a clear sleep plan will assist you to manage your risk as well as ensure that you are providing your body with the rest that it needs every day. What sleep plan will I create and follow to ensure that I have healthy sleep habits?

_____

_____

_____

_____

_____

Problem-Solving

Sometimes people use the Internet as a form of escape. It becomes a way to escape problems, escape negative feelings and/or a way to fill time. As you move away from using the Internet to escape your daily life, you may notice that you simply replace the Internet with other forms of escape such as using alcohol or drugs, reading excessively, engaging in hours of television watching, long hours of playing video games, long periods of daydreaming or working too much. If you are using external means to escape your daily life, what are you avoiding?

Many people have not learned how to resolve problems well. If you grew up in a household where your caregivers did not solve problems effectively, you may lack the skills to deal with certain problems. Expressions such as "Just forget about it", "What will be will be", "Whatever" and "It is what it is" can all be examples of avoidance. Avoidance happens when you have a problem and you decide not to do anything about it. You decide to ignore the problem, minimize the problem, dismiss the problem and/or you generally pretend that the problem does not exist. This does not allow you to resolve outstanding problems.

We often learn how to cope with problems by watching others. Let's explore what worked well and what did not work well in the problem-solving that you observed growing up. Let's reflect on the problems that you and your caregivers and peers faced over the years. This may assist you to address some limitations in your problem-solving skills.

1. What problems did my caregivers face throughout my life?

_____

_____

_____

2. How did my caregivers resolve these problems?

_____

_____

_____

_____

3. What problems did I face as a child?

_____

_____

_____

4. How did my caregivers resolve my problems as a child?

_____

_____

_____

5. What problems did I face as a young adult?

_____

_____

_____

_____

_____

6. How did my peers solve problems?

_____

_____

_____

7. How did I resolve my problems as a young adult?

_____

_____

_____

8. What problems have I faced as an adult?

_____

_____

_____

_____

9. What are the worst ways that I have found to resolve my problems as an adult?

_____

_____

_____

10. What are the best ways that I have found to resolve my problems as an adult?

_____

_____

_____

We all have problems. Some problems are harder to manage than others. Finding appropriate solutions to your problems is essential. When you look over your list of problems, what themes do you notice? What problems have been maintained over time?

Longstanding problems are typically difficult to change. When you face a longstanding problem, it is important to be patient with yourself and to understand that you may have to make repeated efforts to address the entrenched patterns of thoughts and behaviors that you or others may be engaging in that perpetuate the problem.

Joe is a married man. He has a wife, grown kids and pets that he loves. Joe has often struggled with problems in his family life that he has not been able to resolve. He wishes that his wife would be more affectionate toward him. He would like his children to pay more attention to him. Joe has talked about this before to both his wife and his kids. They tell him that everything is fine and not to worry. Sometimes, after he talks to them, they show him more affection. Joe notices that things are better. These changes don't always last. Some days he feels that nothing has really changed. Joe wants to stay in his marriage, and he wants to be a supportive father to his children. Joe is facing a perpetual problem.

When faced with longstanding and seemingly intractable problems you may need to determine how you can adjust if it becomes apparent that a particular situation will not fundamentally change. Some problems won't change, but you can change how you respond to the problem.

Whether you are facing a longstanding and seemingly intractable problem or a problem that is much easier to fix, the steps to effective problem-solving remain the same.[5]

1. Clearly identify the issue.
2. Identify your feelings about the situation or issue.
3. Brainstorm solutions. Make a list of all the possible solutions, no matter how crazy they might first appear to be.
4. Decide on the best solution on your list and try it.
5. Evaluate the outcome of your solution. Did it work? If not, try a different solution to see if a different strategy would work better.

If these steps do not work for you, it is important to ask for help! When solving problems asking for help can be essential. Frequently, others can identify alternative solutions that you may not have considered. This can be particularly useful in situations where you are feeling very emotional about a certain problem.

Ensure that you are not using avoidance and simply ignoring your problems.
Find ways to address your problems.
If you struggle to address your problems, ask for help.
Apply specific problem-solving skills to help you reach your goals!

To improve my problem-solving skills, I will:

_____

_____

_____

_____

_____

_____

_____

_____

Childhood Sexual Abuse

Many people have a history of sexual victimization as a child or youth. The impact and the consequences of being sexually victimized as a child can be long-lasting. For many, there is significant shame associated with experiencing one incident or multiple incidents of sexual abuse as a child or youth. Particularly for males, the shame associated with being sexually abused can be enormous. Being victimized can lead you to feel powerless against others and hopeless about the world around you. The first step in recovery is to address your harmful behaviors toward others. Completing this workbook and focusing on your use of CSEM is a necessary step toward change. As you address your use of CSEM, there is room to address your prior victimization. There are many great books to help victims regain a sense of power and control in their lives. One example of a book geared toward male survivors of sexual abuse is *Evicting the Perpetrator* by Ken Singer. This book is helpful in explaining the pathways toward offending, some of which you may notice within yourself, and/or identify in your own abuser.

Frequently, male survivors of childhood sexual abuse do not identify themselves as being victims of abuse. This can be reflected in beliefs such as "This happens all the time", "I wanted it", "She was much older, so I was lucky to be initiated into sexual activity", "It's not a big deal", "I was chosen because I was special/unique". These beliefs can impact your ability to challenge your own unhelpful thinking patterns. In addition, these beliefs may have been introduced to you and reinforced by your perpetrator, who wished to groom you into engaging in unwanted sexual behaviors without detection to him or herself. One way to explore the impact of your childhood sexual experiences is to evaluate whether or not the sexual behaviors occurred within a legal framework. Were the behaviors illegal? If so, it was sexual abuse. This reflection can have a sobering effect. If the behavior was illegal, the resulting beliefs that you were told, for example "It's Ok", "I know that you liked it", served as grooming strategies rather than accurate information.

Some users of CSEM report that they were searching online for images of the sexual abuse that they experienced and that this led to their initial use of CSEM. Your own fear about the presence of online images related to your sexual victimization is a real concern. Your fear can help you empathize with all victims of CSEM. It is important to remember, however, that the search for such images led others to be victimized in this process. In addition, exposing yourself to unhealthy and harmful images will not assist you to process and resolve your feelings regarding the abuse you experienced. Trying to find particular images on the Internet can be like looking for a needle in a haystack. Also, say you were to find images of yourself – what then? How can this process benefit you? If you know that these images do exist, speak with your local law enforcement authority. This is the best way to help you create a plan to address your concerns about those pictures.

Some people have noticed that the viewing of CSEM provided them with emotional comfort as it confirmed that they were not alone in having been sexually abused. Some experienced mixed feelings of disgust but also feelings of sexual excitement or a sense of emotional closeness to their abuser when thinking about their experience of childhood sexual abuse. Sometimes, the viewing of CSEM feels tempting because it can remind you of those feelings. Clearly, the relationship between childhood sexual abuse and the viewing of CSEM can be complicated. It is important that you address your abuse so that you are less vulnerable to viewing CSEM and so that you can heal.

Did I experience unwanted sexual behaviors as a child or youth? Yes ___/No ___
Did I experience illegal sexual behaviors as a child or youth? Yes ___/No ___
When I think about my unwanted sexual experiences, what feelings do I notice in my body?

_____

_____

_____

_____

When I think about my unwanted sexual experiences, what emotions do I have?

_____

_____

_____

How did my unwanted sexual experiences impact my beliefs about children/youths and sexuality?

_____

_____

_____

What consequences am I still carrying as a result of my unwanted childhood sexual abuse?

_____

_____

_____

There are support groups for both male and female survivors of sexual abuse. In addition, there are many mental health professionals who specialize in interventions aimed at reducing the impact of childhood trauma. Reach out and get assistance if your current treatment provider is not able to address this issue with you. Therapies aimed at helping you resolve childhood trauma should leave you feeling positive, powerful and with increased resilience. Seek an experienced trauma specialist for additional assistance.

CHAPTER SUMMARY

- Sleep matters! Ensure that your sleep habits are positive and resolve any ongoing sleep difficulties.
- Create a plan to stay accountable about your Internet use in the evening and/or at night.
- Identify and resolve your problems.
- Notice your problem-solving strategies and seek to improve these on a regular basis.
- Don't avoid problems; this tends to make things worse, not better!
- Childhood sexual victimization can continue to haunt you. If you have suffered childhood sexual abuse, take the time to address the impact of your own sexual victimization.
- Seek out additional mental health assistance as needed to discuss these themes in more detail.

NOTES

1 Bert, F., Gualano, M. R., Giacomelli, S., Martorana, M., & Siliquini, R. (2018). Are smartphones and tablets influencing the quality of your sleep? An Italian survey. *Epidemiology. Biostat. Public Health*, 15(e12808). https://doi.org/10.2427/12808.

2 Rohsenow, D. J., Howland, J., Arnedt, J. T., Almeida, A. B., Greece, J., Minsky, S., Kempler, C. S., & Sales, S. (2010). Intoxication with bourbon versus vodka: Effects on hangover, sleep, and next-day neurocognitive performance in young adults. *Alcoholism: Clinical and Experimental Research*, 34, 509–518. https://doi.org/10.1111/j.1530-0277.2009.01116.x

3 Herrmann, E. S., Johnson, P. S., Vandrey, R., & Johnson, M. W. (2017). Morning administration of oral methamphetamine dose-dependently disrupts nighttime sleep in recreational stimulant users. *Drug and Alcohol Dependence*, 178, 291–295. https://doi.org/10.1016/j.drugalcdep.2017.05.013

4 Chinoy, E. D., Duffy, J. F., & Czeisler, C. A. (2018). Unrestricted evening use of light-emitting tablet computers delays self-selected bedtime and disrupts circadian timing and alertness. *Physiological Reports*, 6(10), e13692. https://doi.org/10.14814/phy2.13692. PMID: 29845764; PMCID: PMC5974725.

5 Original model developed by E. Schein. For details see Collins, S. B. (2021). *A historical analysis study of Edgar H. Schein and implications for leaders and organization development practitioners* (Order No. 28547264). Available from ProQuest Central; Publicly Available Content Database. (2553475986).

11

Internet Health

CLINICIAN GUIDE

Examining the client's use of the Internet is another cornerstone of CSEM treatment. The Internet and the use of computers is obviously problematic for many who access CSEM. Internet use is both pervasive and problematic for many people. Too many hours online, not being purposeful with our Internet use or using the Internet for entertainment creates difficulties for many of us. In addition, CSEM offenders often have a history of using the Internet to satisfy their non-sexual and sexual needs. Of concern, they sometimes establish negative peer groups online that encourage and promote CSEM use. As such, addressing the client's Internet use is an essential part of the treatment plan.

We first ask the client to reflect on their online use. As many clients are no longer allowed to access the Internet due to criminal justice restrictions, it may be difficult to understand the full extent of their previous Internet use. Discuss how they used the Internet prior to their arrest and/or their CSEM treatment. In particular, ask about the client's use of the Internet for their entertainment, their social connections and their sexuality. It is likely that excessive Internet use was occurring in many other aspects of their lives, not simply as it pertains to their sexuality. It may also be that their use of the Internet has caused other problems in their relationships or that their Internet use has contributed to their social isolation. Whatever the case, start with exploring how they used and/or misused the Internet in the past.

Once the client can outline difficulties in their previous Internet use, it will become easier to define healthy Internet use. For example, clients may identify that their use of the Internet for their sexuality was a celebratory event that occurred every Friday night as a reward for finishing their week, or that it was a regular way to address their sexual needs when they felt aroused or perhaps it was a time filler when they were feeling bored or lonely. Clients might identify that their Internet use was associated to a particular feeling, for example, feeling angry or sad. Once the pattern is identified, they can begin to address their needs in more helpful ways.

Finding alternative activities rather than going online is important. The clinician can help the client determine if it is best to entirely forgo any Internet use or avoid using the Internet for their sexual expression. A third possibility would be to not use the Internet when they are experiencing specific emotional states that they have identified as being risky. We strongly recommend that while using the Internet, clients work with devices that are equipped with accountability software in order to more effectively manage their Internet use.

DOI: 10.4324/9781003388142-12

Why do people find themselves saying and doing things online that they would not do in person? The online world has specific features that impact our perceptions of the online environment, and these effects can impact online behaviors (Suler, 2004; Cheung, Wong, & Chan, 2021; Hills & Argyle, 2003; Hayne & Rice, 1997; Malamuth, Linz, & Weber, 2013; Rimer, 2017). For example, the online environment can result in what has been described as the online disinhibition effect. There are various ways to conceptualize online disinhibition, including: a behavioral impact leading to both benign and toxic disinhibition, a psychological impact leading to users being less restrained online than offline and a recognition that the Internet itself presents with various characteristics that encourage disinhibition as identified by dissociative anonymity, invisibility, asynchronicity, solipsistic introjections, dissociative imagination and minimization of status and authority (Cheung, Wong, & Chan, 2021; Suler, 2004). Rimer (2017) discusses how elements of the online environment, such as distancing, anonymity, detachment and cultural othering can facilitate CSEM use. These characteristics of the Internet may lead to modified boundaries while online (Rimer, 2017). In addition, CSEM users perceived less social enforcement and less surveillance when online (see Rimer, 2017, 2019 for details).

The concept of distancing is included in features of online disinhibition. Distancing can be understood as feeling separate from events that occur online (Rimer, 2017). Given that online content often does not occur in real time and the content appears separate from ourselves when we are online, it can be easier for people to feel distant from the material they are engaging with (Suler, 2004). This may disinhibit CSEM users more particularly as it relates to older, obviously dated images and videos of children. Explore whether the client felt psychologically distant from the material with which they were engaging, or did they perhaps distance themselves while online by using other means such as intoxicants? What can they do to remain more anchored in their own personal identity and values while online?

The concept of invisibility has been argued to result from a person not being physically seen by others when they are online (Suler, 2004). This can lead to people having the courage to go places online that they would not normally go, and you may see a difference between a person's identity and their online behaviors (Suler, 2004; Cheung, Wong, & Chan, 2021). In addition, being online can feel like you are in an anonymous space. This is referred to as *dissociative anonymity* (Cheung, Wong, & Chan, 2021). It is easy to feel alone and "in private" when using a computer, particularly late at night. Also, a person can easily lie about their online identity. It can sometimes be hard to remember that what you do and say online is never private. Ask clients to explore how they felt when they were online. What elements of anonymity did they recognize when they were online?

Detachment involves the belief that the online material is not personally connected to the individual (Rimer, 2017). An example is the belief that the client's behavior is not morally culpable, because they did not create the material and are simply viewing what others have placed on the Internet. This can lead to people taking very little responsibility for the content they are observing while online. In addition, often clients do not know the victims personally, or the victims are part of another ethnic group and/or live in another country. Rimer (2017) describes this process as Cultural Othering. This creates difficulties as clients fail to perceive that victims from other ethnic groups and/or geographic locations are real people with real feelings. To assist clients, focus on making the victims real despite never having met and/or interacted with them.

Other elements associated with the online environment include asynchronicity, solipsistic introjection and dissociative imagination. Asynchronicity reflects the delayed responses that are possible in the online world (Suler, 2004). You engage online with content that has been created in a separate time and space, and you can choose when to engage or disengage with these materials. Solipsistic introjection refers to how online words, ideas and images live in our heads and how we create a voice or a persona that represents these in our minds. This appears to be particularly relevant to written messages. Dissociative imagination is likely a concept that is particularly relevant for the CSEM client group. Dissociative imagination describes how individuals sometimes perceive the online environment as being a world of imagination that has no connection to reality (Cheung, Wong, & Chan, 2021). Ask clients to explore their concept of the online world as it relates to reality, imagination and what they view as real vs not real.

Finally, the lack of perceived enforcement online is referred to as the minimization of authority (Suler, 2004; Cheung, Wong, & Chan, 2021). The lack of online enforcement of pro-social norms and the lack of perceived enforcement in the online environment can impact a person's behavioral choices (Rimer, 2017). Explore the client's perception that the online environment lacks enforcement. If this is an issue for your client, address how they can create online enforcement for themselves; for example, adding a picture of their family on their devices, creating visible reminders and/or using a software accountability program.

As a result of these unique features of the online environment, various boundaries may be more easily breached (Rimer, 2017). Explore facilitating elements of the Internet with the client (see Suler, 2004; Rimer, 2017, 2019 for further discussion of these important themes). The clinician's role is to create an open discussion regarding the pitfalls of the virtual environment and how the environment itself can contribute to risk.

As noted here, there are many ways that the Internet environment can be challenging for clients. Some additional pitfalls that contribute to problematic Internet use are discussed in the client section of this workbook. These include:

- Believing the Internet is private
- Believing if it is online, it must be ok
- Negative online friends
- You never know what you will see
- You think that you can hide
- Time becomes meaningless
- You use it to feel better

The client's online community matters. This chapter includes discussion of the client's Internet community, including who the client socializes with online. As noted in the prior chapter on relationships, the clinician is encouraged to help the client balance their involvement in online communities with real-world social activity. In addition, talking specifically about safe and unsafe online communities is essential. Engaging with prosocial groups both online and in their community will foster better choices. Make sure to address the client's use of the Internet while they are following restrictive criminal justice conditions, as well as how they plan to use the Internet once criminal justice sanctions are no longer in place.

Discussing ways that the client used to avoid detection online is another way to identify issues that may need to be included in their Internet safety plan. They may require more stringent external controls and accountability if they are very enthused by the online environment and/or if they are used to hiding their online activities. Their overall use of technology may be something that they need to discuss with a well-informed accountability partner. We will talk more about how to create and establish accountability plans and an accountability partner in a later chapter.

If you do not feel competent in your understanding and use of technology, we encourage you to learn more about online communities and online environments. This will help you better understand how the client was engaging online and how the client plans to navigate online in the future. Alternatively, ask the client to share their knowledge with you as another way to gain insights about the online environment.

Help the client create an Internet safety plan that is both effective and realistic. Focus on steering the client toward a plan that they will be enthusiastic about applying in their life. Keep the plan focused on as many approach goals as you can. Approach goals involve healthy and satisfying objectives in contrast to avoidance goals that focus on simply restricting choices and behaviors (Elliot & Covington, 2001; Gable, 2006; Elliot, Gable, & Mapes, 2006). Approach goals tend to be more effective for facilitating and sustaining motivation for change.

When discussing the elements of a good Internet safety plan, consider the following:

- Internet access (Location)
  - where in the home will it be safest for online access to occur?
  - what type of device will they use to access the Internet; for example, game consoles, cellphones, tablets, stationary computers, etc.?
- Internet access (Timing)
  - are there times of the day where it is more likely that the client will make poor choices online?
  - is it helpful to focus their Internet use on a specific time of day?
- Internet access (Content)
  - what online activities or online interests are safe? For example, going to look for the answer to a specific question, keeping a calendar, doing their banking or buying tickets for an upcoming show.
  - what online activities or online interests are problematic? For example, follow specific message boards, sending sexual pictures to strangers or being willing to following unknown links online.
- Internet access (Social)
  - what platforms are safe for them?
  - who is safe in the online community?
  - who will they interact with online?
- Internet access (Accountability)
  - Who will be their accountability partner?
  - What software program will they use to better manage their online choices?
  - How will they create accountability online?
  - How will they address common Internet pitfalls?

There may be elements to add to the Internet safety plan that are specific to your client's needs. Please add as many elements as needed to address the client's safe use of the Internet. This plan is designed to address your client's particular risk factors. Focus on creating a plan that is reasonable and specific and addresses the client's needs, while adding as many approach goals as possible and limiting avoidance goals.

Consider your client's favorite sites and online habits. Are they willing to avoid a problematic online community or replace this community with a safer choice? If not already addressed, the Internet safety plan should also identify parameters for their general pornography use. Explore any areas of resistance as it applies to their online environment and the Internet safety plan.

The goal is to create a longstanding management plan for the client that will endure past the end of their criminal justice involvement. Managing their Internet use is important whether this plan will be put in place immediately or when they obtain Internet access in the future due to current criminal justice limitations. Create a plan for future Internet use that works for your client and addresses their risk factors.

REFERENCES

Cheung, C. M. K., Wong, R. Y. M., & Chan, T. K. H. (2021). Online disinhibition: Conceptualization, measurement, and implications for online deviant behavior. *Industrial Management + Data Systems*, *121*(1), 48–64.

Elliot, A. J., & Covington, M. V. (2001). Approach and avoidance motivation. *Educational Psychology Review*, 13(2), 73–92. https://doi.org/10.1023/A:1009009018235

Elliot, A. J., Gable, S. L., & Mapes, R. R. (2006). Approach and avoidance motivation in the social domain. *Personality & Social Psychology Bulletin*, *32*(3), 378–391. https://doi.org/10.1177/0146167205282153

Gable, S. L. (2006). Approach and avoidance social motives and goals. *Journal of Personality*, *74*(1), 175–222. https://doi.org/10.1111/j.1467-6494.2005.00373.x

Hayne, S., & Rice, R. (1997). Attribution accuracy when using anonymity in group support systems. *International Journal of Human Computer Studies*, *47*, 429–450. https://doi.org/10.1006/ijhc.1997.0134

Hills, P., & Argyle, M. (2003). Uses of the Internet and their relationship with individual differences in personality. *Computers in Human Behavior*, *19*, 59–70.

Malamuth, N., Linz, D., & Weber, R. (2013). The internet and aggression: Motivation, disinhibitory, and opportunity aspects. In Yair Amichai-Hamburger (Ed.), *The social net: Understanding our online behavior* (2nd ed.). Oxford Academic. https://doi.org/10.1093/acprof:oso/9780199639540.003.0007

Rimer, J. R. (2017). Internet sexual offending from an anthropological perspective: Analysing offender perceptions of online spaces. *Journal of Sexual Aggression*, *23*(1), 33–45. https://doi.org/10.1080/13552600.2016.1201158

Rimer, J. R. (2019). "In the street they're real, in a picture they're not": Constructions of children and childhood among users of online child sexual exploitation material. *Child Abuse & Neglect*, *90*, 160–173. https://doi.org/10.1016/j.chiabu.2018.12.008

Suler, J. (2004). The online disinhibition effect. *Cyberpsychology & Behavior*, *7*(3), 321–326. https://doi.org/10.1089/1094931041291295

CLIENT WORKBOOK

Learning Objectives

In this chapter, you will:

a) reflect on your use of the Internet
b) reflect on the presence of negative peers online
c) reflect on your use of sex online
d) start outlining your healthy Internet safety plan

The Internet has provided us with an incredible means to communicate. It has opened the world to us. The Internet allows us to pay bills, apply for government services, communicate with friends or family who live far away, learn about other cultures and countries as well as explore geography and other parts of the world that are not easily accessed. In fact, it allows us to learn about a variety of things! Do you need to know how to unclog a sink, fix a motor or find the owner's manual for your new tool? These are all things that you can do online. Unfortunately, the Internet has also brought with it easy access to all things sexual. If you want to explore any sort of sexual activity, legal or illegal, the Internet will provide this to you.

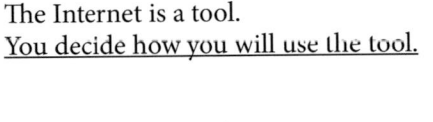

The Internet is a tool.
<u>You decide how you will use the tool.</u>

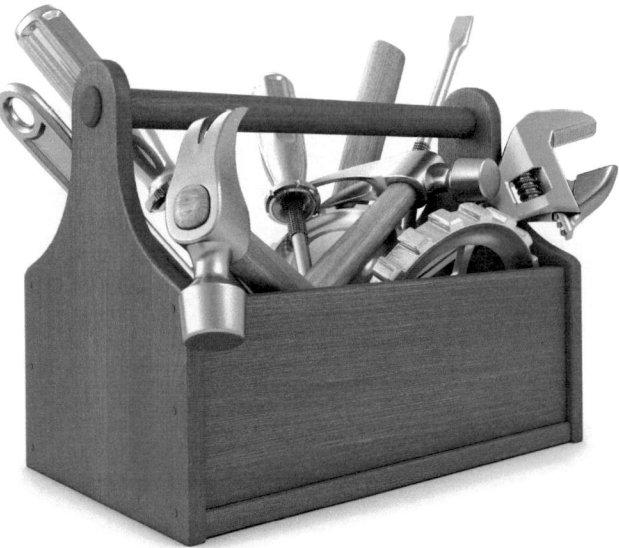

Figure 11.1 The Internet is a tool

The Internet and You

Using the Internet can be very helpful, but there are many ways that you can abuse your time online. Your Internet use can be overly time-consuming. You can spend too many hours online. You can spend too much money online. You can say hurtful things to others online. You can get caught up in social media drama. Some people find themselves using the Internet to cope with negative emotions like feeling lonely, sad, mad or bored. Also, you might find yourself becoming cranky, irritable and moody if the Internet is not available to you. Maybe you have been unsuccessful at reducing your use of the Internet or lost friends, jobs or other opportunities because of your Internet use. These are all indicators of problematic Internet use.

- What is working well and what is not working so well with your use of the Internet?
- What does healthy Internet use look like?

Let's reflect on your behaviors and views about your Internet use.

I use the Internet about _____ hours a day
I believe that it is acceptable to be online about _____ hours a day
I believe that I spend too much time online Y____/N _____
I spend more time online than I want to spend online (0 = never, 100= all the time)
0 . . . . 50 100
Overall, I generally engage in Internet use that is (circle one): healthy or unhealthy

Your beliefs about your Internet use can dictate your behaviors online. Do you think that it is ok to be online at the dinner table? Do you think that it is ok to be online when you are out with friends? Do you think that it is ok to be online when you are at work (for non-work-related activities)? Do you think that it is ok to go online when you are feeling bad after a hard day? Let's reflect on your beliefs about the online world.

　　What do you believe about the online environment? Being online means what to you? Describe your beliefs about the online world.

_____

_____

_____

_____

_____

You may have beliefs like "My online space is private" or "What I do online isn't real, it isn't really me"! Let's look at some of the realities about the online environment.

Internet Pitfalls – Believing the Internet Is Private

Online feels private when you are interacting with a screen alone in your room or when you are interacting with a specific group of people online. In fact, all your activities online can be tracked and are often tracked by many groups. There is more research being done with the tracking information from our online choices. Online is not private. What you do online can be traced back to you. If you are engaging in illegal activities online, you can be found. You can be found even if you are doing things that you believe will keep you hidden online. It is essential that you remember that your online presence is the same as your in-person presence. These are not two different worlds. You are the same person online as you are in person.

How do I present myself online? When I look at my choices online, people will think that I am:

_____

_____

_____

How do I present myself in the real world? When I look at my choices in the real world, people will think that I am:

_____

_____

_____

I want to present myself, both online and in the real world, as a person who is:

_____

_____

_____

Internet Pitfalls – Believing If It's Online It Must Be Ok

The Internet can leave you with the impression that if something is posted online or written online, it is ok. When you see something online, you can start believing that it is normal. For example, "This picture is here so it must be ok" or "People are talking about this, so it must be ok". You can see how this is a thinking error. For example, in life as long as you have the money, you can go and buy as much pizza from the store that you want to buy; does that make eating 20 pizzas ok for you? Is that a good idea? Is it a good choice? Just because something is posted online does not make it ok.

> Pierre is online scrolling through a popular site where people post their thoughts and opinions about many subjects. It can be a great place to get information. Pierre likes learning and he is very curious. He sees a discussion board about people who pretend to be kids when they are online. They do this and then talk about sexual stuff. There is a link to read some of their stories. Pierre decides to click on the link to see what they are talking about. He tells himself that it might be interesting to see what they are saying. If they are talking about it, it must be ok.

When you use the Internet for sexual purposes, things can quickly escalate. There are many illegal sexual themes online. Again, people believe that if it is online, it must be legal. This is not true. While it can be difficult to police the Internet, the fact that material is online does not make it legal. The people you are viewing online are real people. If you are watching someone being abused online, they are being abused. In real life, would you intervene, go for help, call police or would you watch and participate in the abuse? <u>Which choice fits best with who you want to be?</u>

Internet Pitfalls – Negative Online Friends

Who you hang out with matters. It matters a lot. What are the qualities of your online peers?

> Joseph doesn't have many friends. He is lonely. He starts to hang out online with people who think he is funny. They like his jokes and ask him about his day. Joseph notices that they talk to each other about everything and anything. They are not politically correct and say some things that are pretty extreme. Despite this, it is nice to have people to talk to. Over time, the people he is talking to online start talking about sex with kids. They invite him to another chat with more extreme material. Joseph wants to go along; he likes talking to them.

Your online peers matter. If you hang out with people who are doing illegal things online, you will likely be more okay with doing illegal things online. If you hang out with people who think that it is ok to talk about sex with children, you will be exposed to those ideas, and you may start to think that it's okay too. They will seem normal because other people in your group will act like it is normal. Just like the earlier example, if you spend time with people who eat 20 pizzas every Saturday night, this will seem like a reasonable thing to do, even if it is not.

Internet Pitfalls – You Never Know What You Will See

Have you ever noticed that you would never have considered something sexually arousing, but once you saw it online, you started thinking about it more? The dangerous thing with online sex is that once you have seen something, you can't unsee it. Once you have been presented with an idea, you may start considering it. You may start considering things as being sexually arousing that you had not considered in the past. This is why what you view online matters so much!

> Jeffrey received a post on social media from an acquaintance and it said, "Look at this video, man, it is so cool, so hot". Jeffrey has no idea if this is a healthy choice for himself unless he has very good knowledge of the person sending him the information. Should he click on the link?

If you choose to engage sexually online, you must only connect with positive, healthy topics. As you know, that is often hard to do. There are many illegal, harmful or unhealthy sexual topics online. Incest-related images and discussions are a good example. Just because pornography websites post many images, videos and stories involving incest, does that make it legal/healthy for you? You are what you think. <u>Your thoughts matter</u>. Stay away from unhealthy sexual material. If you must use the Internet for sex, only use legal, consensual and healthy sexual material.

<u>Internet monitoring software is available and can be used on all your electronic devices.</u> This software will limit your ability to access violent and/or sexual content. There are various applications that block violent and/or sexual content, accountability programs and parental control software programs. Importantly, this type of software can send accountability reports to your assigned accountability partner. It will track where you go online and send those links to any person you choose. This way, you have a direct line of accountability. It is smart to find an accountability partner who will receive daily reports of where you are going online.

Internet Pitfalls – You Think That You Can Hide

You may be very good with computers, or you may work in a field that involves computers. Computer knowledge may be your strength. This strength can lead you to believe that you do not have to worry about online detection. Making good choices online isn't only about detection. It is about making choices that reduce the sexual exploitation of children. It is about making choices that are positive for the entire community. It is about making choices that lead to your best life. We encourage you to reflect on the following questions:

In the past, what did I do to hide my online behaviors?

_____

_____

_____

_____

_____

How does my online behavior align with my life goals?

_____

_____

_____

_____

Internet Pitfalls – Time Becomes Meaningless

Many people report that they waste a lot of time online. Their productivity goes down and they lose motivation. Sometimes people start turning down invitations to be with their friends or family because they would rather spend their time online. They put all their focus online. They start ignoring things in the real world. They use the Internet to escape their problems, to fill their time or to avoid dissatisfactions in their life.

Searching online without a plan, following each rabbit hole, can lead to spending many, many hours online. Good Internet health means that you are going online only with a specific purpose. For example, "I need to go online to find out how to fix my leaky toilet" or "I need to go online to pay my bills". Many people use the Internet for specific activities quite easily; the difficulty occurs when you are aimlessly looking at links without a purpose. Do you need more specific barriers, such as accessing the Internet in a public place or disconnecting your Wi-Fi router at a specific time each day? Do you need more help to create a positive real-world life for yourself to help you manage your time online?

My plan to manage the amount of time that I will spend online is:

_____

_____

_____

_____

_____

_____

_____

_____

Internet Pitfalls – You Use It to Feel Better

Managing emotions like boredom, anger, loneliness, sadness or discontent by going online is not a helpful strategy. We have talked about the importance of managing your emotions in Chapter 6. We encourage you to review Chapter 6 if you are struggling to manage your emotions or if you are using the Internet to help you manage your emotions.

Does being online feel better than being in the real world? Y ___/N ____
What emotions do I manage by going online?

_____

_____

_____

What can I do to make the real world safer and/or more interesting to me?

_____

_____

_____

_____

Internet Pitfalls – Other

Is there another Internet pitfall that was particularly challenging for you? If so, describe it and then make plan for how you will change it.

_____

_____

_____

_____

_____

_____

Good Internet Health

Your Internet health means that you are using the Internet in ways that are positive and healthy for you. You are interacting with a positive social group, you are not spending too much time online, you have both online and in person friends, you are not using the Internet for sexual purposes and/or you are only using the Internet to access legal material. Your goals when using the Internet are task-based (you are using it to do something specific) rather than avoidance-based (you are using it to aimlessly pass the time or to deal with uncomfortable emotions).

I would describe healthy Internet use as:

_____

_____

_____

_____

I would describe unhealthy Internet use as:

_____

_____

_____

_____

I will know that my Internet use is healthy if I am:

_____

_____

_____

_____

I will know that my Internet use is <u>NOT</u> healthy if I am:

_____

_____

_____

_____

A good Internet safety plan includes very specific goals for your Internet use and a clear plan on how you will stay safe when you are online. Consider the following:

- Internet access (Location)
    ○ Where will you access the Internet?
    ○ What type of device will you use?
    ○ What type of device will you <u>not</u> use?

- Internet access (Timing)
  - When will you access the Internet?
  - When will you <u>not</u> access the Internet?
  - Are there times when it is more likely that you will make poor choices online?
  - Is it helpful to focus your Internet use on different times of the day?
- Internet access (Content)
  - What will you look up online?
  - What are the ways that you will use the Internet?
  - What will you <u>not</u> look up online?
  - What type of entertainment will you seek online?
- Internet access (Social)
  - Who will you talk to online?
  - What platforms will you use online?
  - Who will you <u>not</u> talk to online?
  - What platforms will you <u>not</u> use online?
- Internet access (Accountability)
  - Who will be your accountability partner?
  - What software program will you use to ensure online accountability?
  - How will you address common Internet pitfalls?
  - What type of review of your Internet safety plan will you create to ensure that you stay on track?

I will manage my choices by following a specific plan. My Internet safety plan is:

_____

_____

_____

_____

_____

_____

_____

_____

_____

We will continue to build on your Internet safety plan in Chapter 12. For now, practice your Internet health skills. Do not hesitate to ask for help if you are struggling with your Internet health.

CHAPTER SUMMARY

- Your Internet health is important
- Online is not private!
- Only maintain positive peers online
- Present yourself online in the same way that you present yourself in person
- Reduce your time online
- Use Internet blocking software to block sexual themes online
- Send accountability reports to a trusted person so they can see where you are going when you are online
- Create a healthy Internet safety plan

12

My Safety Plan

CLINICIAN GUIDE

The goal of this chapter is to provide the client with a concise and complete document that they can rely on to manage future risk and risk factors. The entire treatment plan revolves around creating an effective and relevant safety plan for the client. This plan needs to include all the elements and risk factors identified throughout treatment. First, the client will be able to present their understanding of the work they have accomplished throughout the program. Second, the client will be able to create reminders for themselves and put procedures in place to address risk factors that may occur in the future.

An important element to facilitate motivation for change is encouraging the client to move toward positive goals, rather than focusing on behaviors they want to avoid. As such, you want the safety plan to emphasize approach goals. Approach goals are things that the client wants to achieve (Elliot & Covington, 2001; Gable, 2006; Elliot, Gable, & Mapes, 2006). For example, an approach goal of wanting to feel fit and more energetic could result in a decision to begin regularly going to the gym. This is in contrast to wanting to avoid becoming overweight and hence deciding to go to the gym. According to this theory, the individual who focuses on what they will "get" from going to the gym is more likely to continue going in contrast to the one who simply wants to avoid becoming overweight. Another example of an approach goal would be to feel more connected and closer to other people. In this example, a client may decide to join a social group of some type such as a hiking group, a jogging group or an in-person gaming group. Approach goals feel good and have positive effects on the person.

There are other types of strategies to include in the safety plan. These include avoidance goals where necessary, as well as coping strategies and escape strategies. These strategies help the client put limitations in place that they feel are necessary to address their risk in the community. Coping strategies highlight situations that need to be managed in the moment, and escape strategies are situations where the client simply needs to leave immediately. Note that the strategies in the safety plan need to reflect the client's beliefs and opinions about what will help keep them safe. Consistent with the therapeutic model discussed throughout this workbook, explore alternatives with your client that address risk relevant targets and meet their personal preferences, rather than directing your client in creating a plan that suits your beliefs and opinions about what might be best for them.

External and internal barriers create limitations that help the client make better choices. Barriers that are external to the client such as blocking and accountability software, leaving

DOI: 10.4324/9781003388142-13

the computer in a common room as well as the restrictions provided by the criminal justice system create accountability and external structure. Internal barriers are beliefs, thoughts and values that guide decision-making and help people determine what decisions they want to make in accordance with their own value structure. We need both external and internal barriers as part of a safety plan. Some risk factors will be well managed with external structure, and others are best managed within the client's internal structures. When discussing barriers with the client, we suggest that you find barriers that will work best for them. If they tend to be quite defiant, any barriers or restrictions will likely be problematic. In that case, focus more heavily on approach goals and include a reward system to assist with the application of their safety plan. When designing an effective safety plan, there are personal differences; what will work for one person may not work for another person. Use your clinical creativity to assist your client in finding the best strategy.

Encourage the client to identify their longstanding vulnerabilities and their triggers. Reviewing the longstanding vulnerabilities and triggers that were identified earlier in treatment is a good way to ensure that relevant risk factors are included in the safety plan. The safety plan should explicitly identify how each risk factor will be addressed. Go through each risk factor and ensure that every element has a corresponding safety plan in place.

Adding the Internet safety plan created in the previous chapter will allow the client to create a comprehensive plan that addresses sexual self-regulation and the healthy use of the online environment. In this population, addressing both these elements is essential.

In addition, we encourage you to review your clinical file information. This will ensure that you have identified all the risk factors (e.g. longstanding vulnerabilities and triggers) that have been previously discussed. Review past assessments and any other sources of information that speak to the client's risk factors. You were asked to review your file at approximately the mid-point of this workbook; doing it again at the end of treatment is highly recommended. Ensure that the client's safety plan covers all the longstanding vulnerabilities and triggers that were identified throughout treatment. If the client does not agree with a risk factor that you identified, facilitate a discussion to explore that in more detail. Oftentimes, this discussion will clarify the importance of that particular risk factor or address any misunderstandings in your work together. The client can then make the decision to include it, or not, in their plan.

We include a suicide prevention plan as part of the client's overall safety plan. This is one way to ensure that suicide risk has been addressed and also recognizes that the client may experience suicidal thoughts in the future. This may be particularly relevant if they experience rejection in their relationships as a result of their CSEM use becoming known in the community or within their particular social group.

By this point, the client should be able to readily recall and identify their risk factors as well as explain the specific skills and interventions they use to manage those risk factors. You may want to encourage your clients to create a smaller, more summarized version of the safety plan. This may be more manageable for them than the full-length version of the safety plan. We leave it to the clinician to develop a strategy for maintaining the safety plan that best works for the client. There are many creative ways to accomplish this goal. For example, we ask clients to identify the most important interventions of their safety plan and to have this on a separate piece of paper or contained in a separate document. This is one way to create a summarized safety plan. The client can also rotate through their safety plan, focusing on one intervention every quarter to maintain their attention to each risk factor (for example, focus on risk factor A and associated intervention from January to March; focus on risk factor B and associated intervention from April to June; focus on risk factor C and associated intervention from July to September and focus on risk factor D and associated intervention from October to December). There are many ways to assist your client to make maintaining their safety plan and reviewing their treatment goals manageable. Find a way that makes sense to the client.

Safety plans are meant to shift and change over time. These plans are live documents. There is a benefit to reviewing the safety plan on a regular basis. Help the client understand the importance of reviewing their plan and sharing their safety plan with others on a regular basis. Find a structure for the review of the safety plan that will work for your client.

This chapter is the main concluding element of the treatment plan. Completing this chapter means that the client can understand and identify their risk factors. It also means that the client has explored, identified and outlined ways that they will manage their risk factors in the future. Continuing to improve and refine their safety plan is an ongoing process. We will talk more about accountability and the maintenance of treatment gains in the next chapter.

REFERENCES

Elliot, A. J., & Covington, M. V. (2001). Approach and avoidance motivation. *Educational Psychology Review, 13*(2), 73–92. https://doi.org/10.1023/A:1009009018235

Elliot, A. J., Gable, S. L., & Mapes, R. R. (2006). Approach and avoidance motivation in the social domain. *Personality & Social Psychology Bulletin, 32*(3), 378–391. https://doi.org/10.1177/0146167205282153

Gable, S. L. (2006). Approach and avoidance social motives and goals. *Journal of Personality, 74*(1), 175–222. https://doi.org/10.1111/j.1467-6494.2005.00373.x

CLIENT WORKBOOK

Learning Objectives

In this chapter, you will:

a) create a safety plan
b) learn about internal and external barriers to accessing CSEM
c) identify approach and avoidance goals
d) identify coping strategies

It's now time to pull it all together. You have worked very hard to explore various aspects of your lifestyle, your thinking patterns, your relationships and your sexuality. The key to change is continuing to move forward by practicing your new skills regularly. It is also useful to have a safety plan. A safety plan is a document that pulls together all your goals, interventions and plans to maintain these new positive changes in your life.

Why a Safety Plan?

A safety plan is a way to make sure that you have a clear plan of what you will do to stay safe. It is also a way to summarize all your ideas and plans in one place. Safety plans are essential. They allow you to clearly outline, for yourself and for others, how you will stay safe in the future and how you will build your healthy life. Also, when others need to know how you will continue to be safe, your safety plan can help communicate your plan of action to others. It is an agreement with yourself and with your loved ones about your new choices. Your safety plan may be quite simple, or it may have many parts. In this chapter, we will review the elements of a complete safety plan and assist you to create your own plan.

Barriers

Barriers are one way to ensure safe choices. There are external and internal barriers. External barriers are things outside of yourself that make it harder to access illegal images. They will literally get in your way. Internal barriers are thoughts, attitudes, beliefs and values that make it harder for you to maintain your illegal behaviors.

Examples of external barriers are:

- accountability software, software that blocks sexual themes from your devices and documents the websites you visit
- providing your partner or friends access to your computer
- placing your computer in an area where others can see the screen
- providing your partner or roommate control over the Wi-Fi so that they can shut it off if you are overextending your use
- scheduling your Wi-Fi router to shut off every evening at a certain time
- using a cell phone that does not allow access to the internet
- making an agreement with your therapist or treatment group to disclose any breaches of sexual boundaries and/or acknowledge risky behaviors
- using the internet only when under the supervision of a trusted support
- adding a picture of a loved one to your screen saver
- limiting the number of hours that you spend online
- regularly attending a support group or therapy that helps to hold you accountable for your behavior

Examples of internal barriers include:

- your desire to change
- caring about your victims
- feelings of guilt and remorse
- understanding the consequences to victims of sexual assault
- your decision to take care of your family and provide for their needs
- your fear of the legal consequences should you continue to access CSEM
- focusing on the consequences to yourself and to others should you continue to use CSEM
- your ability to reliably identify and replace thinking errors as they arise
- your ability to tolerate uncomfortable emotions
- your ability to manage problematic behaviors
- increased resilience because you are leading a healthier lifestyle

In your safety plan, it is a good idea to have both internal and external barriers to using CSEM. Start with listing your barriers to further CSEM use.

My external barriers:

_____

_____

_____

_____

My internal barriers:

_____

_____

_____

_____

Your safety plan starts with you and what you are willing to do. Do not create a safety plan that you are not willing to follow. Making plans that you are not willing to put in place simply doesn't work. This will ultimately negatively impact your motivation to change. Only put forward elements in your safety plan that you are willing to do.

Bill is working hard to change his behaviors. He has completed most of this workbook and is working with a mental health counselor to help him stay safe and build a healthy life. He now wants to put together his safety plan. Bill wants to do this well. He creates a safety plan that includes never being near a computer alone, going to the gym every day and never masturbating. When Bill talks to his counselor, he is reminded that he lives alone and hates going to the gym. What is wrong with his safety plan?

Bill's plan looks great on paper. The problem is that Bill will likely not follow his plan. He doesn't like the gym. He lives alone at home, so not being alone with a computer means that he will never own a computer or an Internet-capable device of any kind. That doesn't seem realistic. Bill must create a realistic plan for himself given his life circumstances. Just like Bill, your plan must be realistic, and it must be a plan that you will follow. Make sure that your safety plan works for you!

Goals

As you pull together your safety plan, notice that clear, specific goals are important. Make your plan about what you will do. Identify changes that others will notice about you. Make a plan with clear and specific goals. You want others as well as yourself to be able to see the changes that you have made to your thinking patterns, emotional management and your life choices.

We started this workbook by exploring your risk for suicide and asking you to connect with a mental health professional should you feel suicidal. In your safety plan, address your suicide risk. Some examples of ways to manage any future risk for suicide might be to call your local crisis line, contact a counsellor, talk to a friend or family member, go to your local hospital emergency room, talk to your family doctor, go to a public area so that you are not alone, go stay with friends, etc. If you do feel suicidal in the future, how would you manage those feelings?

If I am feeling suicidal, I will:

_____

_____

_____

_____

Vulnerabilities and Triggers

Let's review: Please outline the longstanding vulnerabilities and triggers that you identified earlier in this workbook (see your work in Chapter 3). As your treatment progressed, you may have identified additional longstanding vulnerabilities and triggers.

Examples of longstanding vulnerabilities might be:

- thrill-seeking
- rule-breaking
- passive behaviors in relationships
- frequent conflicts in relationships
- experiencing trauma
- an interest in sexual activity with children
- thinking errors about children and sex
- problematic relationships
- drug and alcohol abuse
- difficulties managing your emotions
- mental health problems
- poor sleep hygiene
- having sexual thoughts about children
- focusing too much on sex
- using sex to deal with emotions

- socializing with teens or youths
- difficulties solving problems
- not understanding the rules of sexual consent

In addition, examples of triggers may include:

- being intoxicated
- feeling bored
- surfing the Internet
- declining an invitation to spend time with friends
- a fight with your spouse
- staying up late at night
- feeling anxious
- feeling sad
- feeling sexually aroused
- telling yourself "Who cares? It doesn't matter", "Fuck it"!

Write your longstanding vulnerabilities and your triggers here. This will give you a good start when crafting your safety plan. It is important that your safety plan address all the longstanding vulnerabilities and triggers that are relevant to you. You will use this list to complete your safety plan here.

My longstanding vulnerabilities:

1) _____

_____

2) _____

_____

3) _____

_____

4) _____

_____

5) _____

_____

6) _____

_____

7) _____

_____

8) _____

_____

9) _____

_____

10) _____

_____

My triggers:

1) _____

_____

2) _____

_____

3) _____

_____

4) _____

_____

5) _____

_____

6) _____

_____

7) _____

_____

8) _____

_____

9) _____

_____

10) _____

_____

A complete safety plan allows you to outline barriers as well as coping strategies. While you may do a great job using barriers, you will also need to manage or cope with various situations. Many times, things happen in life that are outside our control. You need to be able to react to situations as they occur. Coping strategies are essential because they help you manage your emotions, thinking and behaviors. Coping strategies also help you manage unpredictable situations. A good safety plan helps you to stay safe in many situations.

The first and most important part of your safety plan involves the positive things that you want in your life. Focusing on positives makes it more likely that you will do these things. Remember Charles from Chapter 5 on Sexual Management? Charles observed that he would masturbate in the morning to get himself going at the start of his day. He joined a running group in the mornings, as it provided him with a sense of purpose and provided a sense of well-being. This is called an <u>approach goal</u>. Approach goals involve emotional, physical and social pursuits that we find inherently attractive and rewarding. These things give us joy, satisfaction, energy and drive. Approach goals work well because we actually WANT to do them. If you are trying to make positive changes in your life, having lots of approach goals will work better than focusing on all the things that you are trying to avoid. Achieving healthy approach goals will also help you manage urges to engage in illegal behaviors, such as accessing CSEM.

Eddie wants to feel better about his body, and he knows that he should avoid eating pastries and cake to reach his goals. But the more he tells himself to avoid eating pastries and cake, the more he wants to eat them. Eddie noticed that he was feeling resentful and irritated because he was giving up something that he wanted. Eddie went to see a counsellor, who told him that it would be more helpful if he focused on doing the things that he likes to do that will bring him closer to his goals. Eddie likes going to the gym because of the good feeling he gets from working out. He likes attending yoga because he likes the sense of calm it provides him. He decides to take a cooking class to help him learn to prepare healthy and tasty food. This satisfied his desire to eat tasty food that also provided him with a sense of satisfaction. Focusing on the things that he liked to do helped Eddie not only feel good about himself but have a life that he found to be more rewarding and satisfying. Within a few months, Eddie noticed how good he was feeling about his body.

When you reflect on your CSEM use, what approach goals would keep you safe and happy? What approach goals would keep you away from using illegal sexual images?
Examples of approach goals might be:

- new leisure activities
- time with friends
- new relationships
- setting good boundaries with others
- exercise
- setting physical fitness goals
- work-related goals
- sticking to a schedule
- better sleep hygiene

What approach goals do you want to set for yourself?
My approach goals include:

1) _____

_____

2) _____

_____

3) _____

_____

4) _____

_____

5) _____

_____

6) _____

_____

As much as we want to focus on approach goals, there are some situations that you simply must avoid. <u>Avoidance goals</u> involve situations, places, thoughts or behaviors that you must avoid. Avoiding things that would increase your risk is an important part of your safety plan.

Examples of avoidance goals are:

- not agreeing to babysit or offering to babysit children
- avoiding partners who have children
- avoiding social gatherings where the focus is on children's activities
- not viewing sexual websites
- not accessing Internet sites that cater to children or that post children's content
- not masturbating to CSEM images in your mind
- not socializing online with strangers or unknown peers
- avoiding unhealthy partners and/or bad relationships
- not staying up late at night
- avoiding drug or alcohol use

What are your avoidance goals?

My avoidance goals include:

1) _____

_____

2) _____

_____

3) _____

_____

4) _____

_____

5) _____

_____

6) _____

_____

Coping Strategies

There are some situations that you simply have to cope with. These situations are managed using your <u>coping strategies</u>. Coping strategies help get you through a tough situation. They allow you to stay in the moment while managing your feelings and thoughts in a positive way.
   Examples of situations where you might use your coping strategies include:

- managing your emotions when you feel sad or lonely
- maintaining a job that you don't necessarily like
- seeing children at a store
- being single when you would prefer to be in a relationship
- dealing with the loss of friends or family members because of your CSEM use
- managing relationships where the trust has been broken due to your CSEM use
- dealing with the legal system if you have been arrested for your actions
- dealing with an urge to masturbate when you are feeling sad, lonely or when you have had a sexual thought about CSEM

You must cope with these situations by finding ways to make the best of the situation and staying on a positive path for yourself. You have the ability to make good choices despite the situation that you are in. How do you plan to cope with difficult situations?
   My coping strategies are:

1) _____

_____

2) _____

_____

3) _____

_____

4) _____

_____

5) _____

_____

6) _____

_____

7) _____

_____

8) _____

_____

9) _____

_____

10) _____

_____

Situations that I will have to cope with in the future are:

1) _____

_____

2) _____

_____

3) _____

_____

4) _____

_____

5) _____

_____

6) _____

_____

7) _____

_____

8) _____

_____

9) _____

_____

10) _____

_____

I will deal with these specific situations by doing:

1) _____

_____

2) _____

_____

3) _____

_____

4) _____

_____

5) _____

_____

6) _____

_____

7) _____

_____

8) _____

_____

9) _____

_____

10) _____

_____

Escape Strategies

Escape is a way to remove yourself from dangerous situations. When you need to escape, often it is because you have gotten much too close to offending. You have moved to a point that is dangerous for yourself and/or others. Escape is your way out! When you were in school, you practiced fire drills that included planning how to get out of the school; those were escape strategies. It is important to have escape strategies in regard to CSEM, sexual attraction to children and/or other risky situations.

Some examples of escape strategies include:

- leaving social events if you find yourself wanting to engage in a sexual interaction with a child who is there
- walking away from your computer
- throwing a device out
- locking a device away for a period of time
- giving your devices to a friend
- going to stay with a friend for a few days
- leaving your home and going for a walk
- throwing out your car keys if you are planning to go buy a prohibited electronic device
- breaking your computer if you are in the midst of searching for illegal images
- going for a run
- leaving when an argument is escalating to violence

Escape when you need to move quickly away from a dangerous situation. Remember that by getting rid of your electronic devices, you ensure that you won't have access to CSEM. It is easy to break an electronic device or to drop it in water in order to disable the device. If you get close to re-offending, what are your escape strategies? What would you do if you were getting too close to returning to CSEM use?

My escape strategies are:

1) _____

_____

2) _____

_____

3) _____

_____

4) _____

_____

5) _____

_____

6) _____

_____

7) _____

_____

8) _____

_____

9) _____

_____

10) _____

_____

Potential situations where I may have to escape in the future:

1) _____

_____

2) _____

_____

3) _____

_____

4) _____

_____

5) _____

_____

6) _____

_____

7) _____

_____

8) _____

_____

9) _____

_____

10) _____

_____

I will escape from these specific situations by doing:

1) _____

_____

2) _____

_____

3) _____

_____

4) _____

_____

5) _____

_____

6) _____

_____

Review

There are many factors that you may have identified as part of your list of longstanding vulnerabilities and triggers. Consider the general problems you were facing at the time of your offending. They may include mental health difficulties, specific personal difficulties, sleep difficulties, problem-solving difficulties, etc. Let's start with reviewing the general problems in your life and identify strategies to address these problems moving forward.

My longstanding vulnerabilities and triggers are:

1) _____

_____

2) _____

_____

3) _____

_____

4) _____

_____

5) _____

_____

6) _____

_____

7) _____

_____

8) _____

_____

9) _____

_____

10) _____

_____

I will better manage my longstanding vulnerabilities and triggers by:

1) _____

_____

2) _____

_____

3) _____

_____

4) _____

_____

5) _____

_____

6) _____

_____

7) _____

_____

8) _____

_____

9) _____

_____

10) _____

_____

Let's review your computer use as it relates to your safety plan. It is important that your safety plan specifically address your computer use. In Chapter 3, we discussed your computer use and CSEM. We also talked about your permission-giving thoughts about using online sexual images in Chapter 7. We discussed Internet health in Chapter 11, and you outlined an Internet safety plan.

Examples of a computer problem might be:

- using a computer alone
- not using accountability software
- using a computer rather than socializing with friends and family
- using a computer to deal with uncomfortable emotions
- not believing that online images involve real people
- using a computer late at night

What longstanding vulnerabilities and triggers did you identify regarding your computer use?

My longstanding vulnerabilities and triggers related to my computer use are:

1) _____

_____

2) _____

_____

3) _____

_____

4) _____

_____

5) _____

_____

6) _____

_____

7) _____

_____

8) _____

_____

9) _____

_____

10) _____

_____

Barriers I will use to better manage my computer use moving forward:

1) _____

_____

2) _____

_____

3) _____

_____

4) _____

_____

5) _____

_____

6) _____

_____

7) _____

_____

8) _____

_____

9) _____

_____

10) _____

_____

In addition to the safety plan elements listed here, it is important to specifically address your sexual behaviors in your safety plan. Whether you clearly outlined longstanding vulnerabilities and triggers related to sex or whether you do not believe that sexuality played a large part in your behaviors, having a plan that includes your sexuality is essential. It is important to review your plan to address your sexuality moving forward. Explore your plan specifically as it relates to your sexuality.

My longstanding vulnerabilities and triggers related to my sexuality are:

1) _____

_____

2) _____

_____

3) _____

_____

4) _____

_____

5) _____

_____

6) _____

_____

Barriers I will use to better manage my sexuality moving forward:

1) _____

_____

2) _____

_____

3) _____

_____

4) _____

_____

5) _____

_____

6) _____

_____

Outlining your thinking errors and/or permission-giving thoughts has been an important part of this workbook. Your thinking matters. Whether you are managing your unhelpful thoughts in general or managing specific thoughts about children and sex, it is essential to maintain healthy thinking patterns. General thinking errors such as "No one likes me", "I am unlovable", "I am useless", "They are all against me" or "I must have it my way" will impact your mood and your ability to manage your emotions. Sexual thinking errors such as "This is a victimless crime", "No one got hurt", "I didn't do anything wrong", "Youths like to expose their bodies online", "They wanted me to use their pictures in this way" or "It's not a real child" will continue to allow you to justify your illegal behaviors and your illegal choices. Both types of thinking patterns need to be better managed. You have already worked on identifying and challenging your unhelpful thoughts. Write down your main thinking errors and the associated replacement thoughts as they relate to your CSEM use. Use an extra sheet of paper if you require more space.

The thinking errors/permission-giving thoughts that led me to use CSEM are:

1) _____

_____

2) _____

_____

3) _____

_____

4) _____

_____

5) _____

_____

6) _____

_____

7) _____

_____

8) _____

_____

9) _____

_____

10) _____

_____

11) _____

_____

12) _____

_____

My replacement thoughts for these thinking errors are:

1) _____

_____

2) _____

_____

3) _____

_____

4) _____

_____

5) _____

_____

6) _____

_____

7) _____

_____

8) _____

_____

9) _____

_____

10) _____

_____

11) _____

_____

12) _____

_____

Your relationships have also been an important focus in this workbook. Relationships can move us toward positive or negative choices. Relationships, both online and in the community, can impact your ability to avoid CSEM and to build a healthy and satisfying life. Looking specifically at your relationships, what have you noticed? What needs to change for you to be satisfied and content in your relationships? What relationship goals do you have moving forward?

My longstanding vulnerabilities and triggers related to my relationships are:

1) _____

_____

2) _____

_____

3) _____

_____

4) _____

_____

5) _____

_____

6) _____

_____

7) _____

_____

8) _____

_____

9) _____

_____

10) _____

_____

My current relationships include:

1) _____

_____

2) _____

_____

3) _____

_____

4) _____

_____

5) _____

_____

6) _____

_____

7) _____

_____

8) _____

_____

I will improve my relationships in the future by:

1) _____

_____

2) _____

_____

3) _____

_____

4) _____

_____

5) _____

_____

6) _____

_____

7) _____

_____

8) _____

_____

It is important to create a safety plan that will be useful to you. In addition, your safety plan needs to be relatively SIMPLE. Many people create elaborate safety plans that do not help because they are confusing, too long and involve too many life changes at once. We ask you to include the top 3 strategies to keep you safe. This section is the shortcut, or the most important things that you need to do to stay safe. Whether these strategies are done daily, weekly or represent a new way of living, it is essential that you boil down your safety plan to a few key ideas so that you do not get overwhelmed and lose sight of the most important elements for maintaining change.

What are the most important changes that you have put in place and maintained throughout your work in this workbook? What are your top few strategies to stay safe?

1) _____

_____

2) _____

_____

3) _____

_____

Safety Plan Examples

Before we pull together your full safety plan, we will look at some examples of other safety plans. It helps to identify similar patterns in others when we are trying to outline our own difficulties. In these examples, notice what fits well for you and what might be different. What will work better for you?

Adam is completing his safety plan. Throughout this workbook, he has identified the following longstanding vulnerabilities: conflicted feelings about his history of childhood sexual abuse, history of drug and alcohol abuse, history of poor relationships, anger problems and a tendency to engage in rule-breaking.

Adam noted that his triggers to CSEM use were: drinking and using drugs, conflicts in his relationships and using masturbation to feel better. Adam's internal barriers are: he is afraid of being arrested and he does not want to let down his family and friends who are starting to trust him again.

Adam's external barriers are: using a software program on all his computer devices, not using the computer in the evening, sticking to his schedule, going to counseling to discuss his history of childhood sexual abuse and attending meditation classes. He has improved his ability to manage his emotions.

Adam can now challenge his various permission-giving thoughts and thinking errors. He knows that the children and youth depicted in CSEM are harmed by his behavior. His plan is to improve his mental health by going for walks, meditating, seeing a therapist, reading more self-help books, keeping a journal and exercising when he is feeling bad. His plan to address his computer use is to keep the software blockers on, send accountability reports to his trusted friend, not to use the computer at night, staying busy and not using the computer for sex. His sexual plan is to find a healthier relationship, only masturbate when he is horny and to never allow himself to fantasize about children and sex. His relationship plan involves finding a new partner with whom he has more in common, a partner that he likes, and to spend more time with his friends. He has not thought about suicide and does not need a suicide plan. He plans to escape any situation where drugs or alcohol are offered and his "no thank you" is ignored or he is feeling pressured to use by others. He is practicing his breathing, meditation and mindfulness skills daily. He plans to cope with being online and not using sexual material by getting up and taking breaks when he is online and not going online if he is feeling horny, lonely or bored. Adam's top three strategies to maintain his changes are to go to the gym daily, stay off the computer at night and to see his friends and family for outings at least once a week and ideally twice a week. Adam feels like he can maintain these changes and is feeling good about moving forward with his plan.

Tom is working on his safety plan. He is struggling to identify things that he can change. Tom identified the following longstanding vulnerabilities: difficulty making friends, tendency to isolate, his dislike of sharing his emotions with others and his lack of computer knowledge.

Tom's triggers are: the death of his wife, being alone most of the time, believing that what he did online was private, loneliness, boredom and feeling sad.

Tom's internal barriers are: his fear of what people would think of him if they found out he was viewing CSEM.

Tom's external barriers are adding a software blocker on his computer and getting a cellphone that does not have access to the internet.

Tom is struggling because he is still very lonely. He misses his wife and can't change the fact that she is gone. He doesn't believe that anyone else would want to be in a relationship with him. He obtained a simple flip phone that does not have access to the Internet. He feels confident that he can rely on his software blocker so that he can use his computer to pay his bills. His plan to address his mental health is to start attending grief counseling and to go to his local coffee shop to read his books. His plan to address his computer use is to only use his computer for a maximum of 2 hours a day. Otherwise, he will watch TV or go do another activity. His plan to address his relationships is still unclear. Tom would like to make some friends, but he is not sure how to go about it. He decides to attend the local seniors' center to participate in their activities 3 times a week. His plan to address his sexuality is to stop using the computer to masturbate. Tom does have some thoughts of suicide and has put the number for the local crisis line on his fridge. He has also decided to talk to his grief counselor about his suicidal thoughts so that they can create a plan to get him reconnected to the community. He will escape situations where he is feeling sad and lonely by calling the crisis line or going to the local coffee shop, as he finds simply being around other people helps him feel less lonely. He will start coping with his feelings by talking with his grief counselor. He will avoid any situations that trigger his grief, like visiting his wife's favorite restaurant. His main strategies to avoid CSEM use involves dealing with his grief, interacting more with others during the week and limiting his computer use.

Mike has many triggers that involve a sexual interest in children. Mike has identified the following longstanding vulnerabilities: years of using pornography to masturbate, a tendency to use all types of pornography, a sexual interest in children and youths and allowing himself to fantasize about children and sex.

Mike identified triggers such as being alone at home, being bored, feeling angry, seeing youths having fun at the local park and feeling like a failure.

Mike's internal barriers include: wanting to avoid any future criminal justice involvement and reminding himself that he feels badly about himself when he does use CSEM. He wants to avoid any police contact.

Mike's external barriers include: ongoing monitoring by the criminal justice system, a prohibition from accessing the Internet, and his family's agreement to intervene if they observe any risky behaviors.

Mike plans to address his sexuality by talking about his interest in children with his therapist, keeping a daily masturbation and sexual fantasy log, curtailing any sexual fantasies that involve children, masturbating less and trying to find adult sexual partners. Mike will address his relationships by practicing his social skills with adults, trying new leisure activities and not approaching children or youths for conversations. Mike will address his computer use by not using computers. When he is allowed to use computers in the future, Mike will use software blocking technology and send accountability reports to his trusted supports. He will avoid any sites that involve children or sites that target children. He will only use the computer for work, to pay bills and to apply for government benefits. Mike plans to have someone with him when he is online. Mike will address his general risk factors by improving his sleep hygiene by not staying up late and going to bed on time; he will reduce his free time by working more hours; he will practice being more assertive when he is talking to others and improve his ability to interact with adults. Mike will take advantage of his criminal justice involvement by talking openly to his community supervisor about his goals and his struggles. He will escape any situations where he notices children or youths are in attendance. He plans to cope with his situation by reaching out to community groups such as Virtuous Pedophiles, b4uact.org, talkingforchange.ca and/or other online supports. Mike will also avoid skate parks, public pools, movie theaters and other places where he used to interact with younger people. Mike's top strategies to address his risk include not engaging in any sexual fantasies involving children, not approaching or talking to children in the community, never being alone with children and not using a computer for sexual stimulation.

Now it is your turn. Let's look at your safety plan in detail:

My Safety Plan

My longstanding vulnerabilities and my triggers:

1) _____

_____

2) _____

_____

3) _____

_____

4) _____

_____

5) _____

_____

6) _____

_____

7) _____

_____

8) _____

_____

9) _____

_____

10) _____

_____

My external barriers:

1) _____

_____

2) _____

_____

3) _____

_____

4) _____

_____

5) _____

_____

6) _____

_____

7) _____

_____

8) _____

_____

9) _____

_____

10) _____

_____

My internal barriers:

1) _____

_____

2) _____

_____

3) _____

_____

4) _____

_____

5) _____

_____

6) _____

_____

7) _____

_____

8) _____

_____

9) _____

_____

10) _____

_____

If I am feeling suicidal, I will:

1) _____

_____

2) _____

_____

3) _____

_____

4) _____

_____

5) _____

_____

My approach goals are:

1) _____

_____

2) _____

_____

3) _____

_____

4) _____

_____

5) _____

_____

6) _____

_____

My coping strategies are:

1) _____

_____

2) _____

_____

3) _____

_____

4) _____

_____

5) _____

_____

6) _____

_____

My escape strategies are:

1) _____

_____

2) _____

_____

3) _____

_____

4) _____

_____

5) _____

_____

6) _____

_____

I will manage my general mental health concerns, longstanding vulnerabilities and triggers by:

1) _____

_____

2) _____

_____

3) _____

_____

4) _____

_____

5) _____

_____

6) _____

_____

7) _____

_____

8) _____

_____

I will manage my computer use by:

1) _____

_____

2) _____

_____

3) _____

_____

4) _____

_____

5) _____

_____

6) _____

_____

7) _____

_____

8) _____

_____

I will manage my sexuality by:

1) _____

_____

2) _____

_____

3) _____

_____

4) _____

_____

5) _____

_____

6) _____

_____

7) _____

_____

8) _____

_____

I will manage my relationships by:

1) _____

_____

2) _____

_____

3) _____

_____

4) _____

_____

5) _____

_____

6) _____

_____

7) _____

_____

8) _____

_____

The replacement thoughts for my thinking errors/permission-giving thoughts are:

1) _____
   _____

2) _____
   _____

3) _____
   _____

4) _____
   _____

5) _____
   _____

6) _____
   _____

7) _____
   _____

8) _____
   _____

9) _____
   _____

10) _____
   _____

Other important aspects of my safety plan:

_____
_____
_____
_____

_____

_____

_____

My top 3 strategies to maintain my changes will be:

1)   _____   _____
2)   _____   _____
3)   _____   _____
4) Optional   _____   _____

Now review your safety plan. Are all your longstanding vulnerabilities and triggers addressed in your safety plan? If not, add them in. Ensure that all the areas that may have been related to your online use of CSEM have been addressed in your safety plan.

I have reviewed my safety plan. All my longstanding vulnerabilities and triggers listed here have been addressed Yes_____ No_____

If your answer is No, what do you need to add to your safety plan? Make a list.

1) _____

_____

2) _____

_____

3) _____

_____

4) _____

_____

5) _____

_____

6) _____

_____

7) _____

_____

8) _____

_____

Add these elements to your safety plan here. It may help to create a final version of your safety plan that you type out and post somewhere visible for yourself as well as share with your supports. This safety plan is a way to remind yourself of your goals and your responsibilities. Make this safety plan a part of your lifestyle moving forward.

It is important to maintain your gains! This can't be overstated. Part of your safety plan should include reviewing the information in this workbook on a regular basis to avoid slipping back into old patterns. In fact, while people can be very motivated to change at first, small slips can lead to bigger slips over time.

> Jeff has worked very hard and taken this workbook seriously. He has made many changes to his life. He no longer accesses online sexual material. He no longer uses CSEM. Jeff has been doing well for 6 months. Slowly, Jeff notices that his mood is lower. He is getting down. He hasn't been able to find a group of friends that make him happy. Jeff is starting to sleep in, he is masturbating more, and he is feeling lonely. Jeff notices this slip. He decides to review this workbook and his safety plan. He also decides to post his safety plan on his fridge. By doing this, Jeff got reconnected to his goals, and he was able to get back on track. He tried some new social events and decided to stop masturbating for a brief period. He also decided to attend a community support group if he notices another slip in the next few months.

Like Jeff, you may experience slips moving forward. It is important to stay positive during these slips. Giving up can lead to a decision to return to CSEM use. Often, giving up is a key turning point back to where you started. Notice words like "Fuck it", "I don't care", "It doesn't matter" and "It's too hard". These words indicate that your motivation has dropped, and you may be thinking about giving up. This is a signal that rapid action is needed to address your treatment engagement. Seek out friends, accountability partners or your support team. They can help you get back on track.

Remember that your success does matter! Your life matters and the choices that you make will lead you to being happier in the future. Alternatively, your choices can lead to feeling sad and regretful in the future. While slips happen, they don't have to take you down. Use your safety plan to keep yourself and others safe.

I will review my safety plan and ensure that I don't slip by doing the following:

1) _____

_____

2) _____

_____

3) _____

_____

4) _____

_____

5) _____

_____

6) _____

_____

Signs that I am slipping include:

1) _____

_____

2) _____

_____

3) _____

_____

4) _____

_____

5) _____

_____

6) _____

_____

Signs that others will notice that I am slipping include:

1) _____

_____

2) _____

_____

3) _____

_____

4) _____

_____

5) _____

_____

6) _____

_____

If I slip, I will contact:

1) _____

_____

2) _____

_____

3) _____

_____

4) _____

_____

Review this chapter on a regular basis to ensure that your plan is working. Post your plan and strategies to avoid slipping in places where you will see them regularly. Remind yourself of your goals!

Your safety plan is a live document. This means that it will change over time. Make sure that you update your safety plan as things in your life change and as you move toward your goals. Updating your safety plan means that you will be actively evaluating your risk, making good choices and solving problems as they come up. This is a great strategy for staying safe!

Don't forget to get others involved in your safety plan. Asking for help, sharing your plans and staying focused on your goals can be great way to stay on track! Accountability partners will be discussed in more detail in the Chapter 12.

CHAPTER SUMMARY

- Your safety plan is an important document
- Create your safety plan
- Include coping strategies, barriers and your longstanding vulnerabilities and triggers in your safety plan
- Review your safety plan regularly
- Use escape strategies to help you get out of risky situations
- Slips can happen. If they do, stay positive and reconnect with your goals to avoid any further CSEM use

13

Accountability

CLINICIAN GUIDE

This final chapter explores the importance of accountability and the maintenance of treatment progress. As noted previously, maintenance is the supportive process that follows treatment. This process allows the client to receive ongoing support with a goal to maintain treatment gains. Maintenance is one way to ensure that there is an ongoing effort to manage risk and to develop a healthier life.

Maintenance can be provided in a variety of ways. For some people, group maintenance programs may be helpful as they provide social interactions, more people to challenge the client should their behaviors slide over time and they provide a community-focused approach to managing risk. Other clients prefer to work on their maintenance plan using an individual approach. Throughout maintenance, clients may start to address other issues such as trauma therapy, general life concerns or other aspects of their personal functioning that could be improved in their quest to maintain a good life.

In this chapter, the clinician is tasked with discussing the client's accountability. How will they be accountable to the significant people in their life? How will they create a supportive team for themselves in their community? Accountability is about sharing the secret of their CSEM use with trusted supports. Accountability is about asking for help and being honest about their CSEM use. Start by encouraging the client to create a network of social supports that will assist them. Creating accountability means relinquishing the secrets involved in their past behaviors and disclosing their struggles with CSEM use. It also involves discussing their current psychological functioning. Work with the client to explore the importance of sharing this problem with others in their lives.

Should the client not be willing to share their CSEM use with at least a few social supports, it would be important to discuss this decision and explore how the client would like to be held accountable in the community. As the mental health professional, you are able to offer some accountability; however, ultimately, the client's accountability is best achieved when it is provided by their family members, close friends and/or their community. As discussed in the previous chapter on relationships, ensuring that the accountability partner is prosocial and helpful is essential. An unhelpful accountability partner or someone who is ultimately encouraging poor choices is not a positive contribution to the goal of building a good life. In addition, ensuring that the proposed accountability partner has the time available to offer support and clarifying the parameters of the support which can be offered will also be important. Discussing potential accountability partners and evaluating their influence, either

DOI: 10.4324/9781003388142-14

positive or negative, as well as their expectations about the accountability partner is one way to address this issue.

For some clients, finding an accountability partner is unrealistic and/or it is not something that the client is willing to do. Such clients may prefer finding social support and accountability by attending a community-based group, such as those found through faith-based groups, Sex Addicts Anonymous or Sexaholics Anonymous groups or other supportive groups available in their community.

We encourage taking the time to review consequences to victims. For some clients, their understanding of consequences is clear, and they are easily able to explore and describe consequences to their victims. For other clients, this may be more difficult. If the client would benefit from a review of the harm that results from accessing CSEM for both themselves and victims, it is recommended that this be reviewed.

Clients are also encouraged to begin to focus their energy on rebuilding trust in their relationships. For family members, partners and close friends who are choosing to remain connected to the client, there will be significant trust building required. This is an essential part of moving through the treatment phase and into the maintenance phase. Trust is built slowly. It relies on good decision-making. Helping the client explore how they would like to rebuild trust in their relationships is an important part of this chapter. <u>Seeking forgiveness is not the goal of trust building</u>. We encourage the client to provide stable, safe and positive interactions with others and to consistently make good choices as a way to repair trust over time. Reminding the client that trust is rebuilt slowly, with time, by consistently making trustworthy choices and engaging in trustworthy actions, along with allowing people to express their feelings of fear, disbelief or concern about their risk is an ongoing part of this process.

This is also the time to ensure that there are no other additional topics to explore as part of the client's treatment plan. Reflect on your client's progress and how they are managing their longstanding vulnerabilities, their triggers and their accountability in the community. If there is an issue that requires attention and exploration, it can be added to the treatment plan at this time.

Creating an accountability plan with the client is one way to re-establish community supports. This plan also serves to reduce the client's use of secrecy. Encourage the client to create and maintain positive supports in the community.

CLIENT WORKBOOK

Learning Objectives

In this chapter, you will:

a) learn about the importance of accountability partners
b) reflect on the impact of your CSEM use on your family and friends
c) recall how victims are impacted by your viewing of CSEM
d) learn about how you can rebuild trust in relationships

Congratulations on your work progressing through this workbook! You have likely made many changes to your life. We hope that you are enjoying an improved lifestyle and an avoidance of CSEM. In this chapter, we will explore themes related to accountability and your relationship with loved ones. There have been many consequences, both for yourself and for others. Let's explore how your relationships can assist you to remain offense-free.

Accountability

Being accountable means being responsible. Whether you are responsible to yourself, a pet, your immediate family members, your friends, your employer, your extended family members and/or your community, you are accountable to someone. Your accountability is both to yourself and to others. Accountability helps you make good decisions. Being accountable to others allows you to think about your decisions before making them. Hopefully, you will continue to make decisions that are in your best interests and the best interests of your community.

Who am I accountable to? Check all that apply.

Myself _____

My children _____

My spouse _____

My friends _____

My family _____

My pets _____

My employer _____

My community _____

Other _____

Other _____

Reflecting on the consequences to others before you make a decision can help change your behavior. What are the consequences to yourself and to others if you use CSEM?

If I choose to use CSEM, the consequences to me would be:

1) _____

_____

2) _____

_____

3) _____

_____

4) _____

_____

5) _____

_____

6) _____

_____

7) _____

_____

8) _____

_____

9) _____

_____

10) _____

_____

If I choose to use CSEM, the consequences to others would be:

1) _____

_____

2) _____

_____

3) _____

   _____

4) _____

   _____

5) _____

   _____

6) _____

   _____

7) _____

   _____

8) _____

   _____

9) _____

   _____

10) _____

   _____

Accountability Partners

Focusing on accountability to help manage your risk just makes sense. That being said, it is important to consider who will actually hold you accountable. Some people in your life will be able to hold you accountable, while others will not. Have you ever had the experience of asking someone to help you change a bad habit? Some people are really helpful; they remind you of your goals, ask you how you are doing and organize social activities to help you stay away from your bad habits. They are also willing to confront you with difficult feedback. These people are great accountability partners! In contrast, other people avoid giving you difficult feedback, they make you feel bad about your goals, they complain about how your efforts are negatively impacting them, they keep offering you temptations, they engage in behaviors that encourage your bad habits and they seem to take satisfaction in your failures. They may even become upset if you are successful in reaching your goals! Such individuals are not helpful accountability partners.

Choose a good accountability partner for you. Share your self-management plan with them. Provide them with information about your emotions log, fantasy logs and thinking errors related to your CSEM use. Discuss the factors that have preceded your CSEM use. Explain your future goals. Ask this accountability partner to help keep you on track. Ask them to provide you with honest feedback about areas of concern. Schedule set meeting times to discuss and review your progress. Identify when you can contact your accountability partner for additional help as needed (for example, is your accountability partner available 24/7 or only on Saturday mornings?). Ensure that you are both comfortable with your roles in your accountability relationship.

A good accountability partner for me would have these qualities:

1) _____

_____

2) _____

_____

3) _____

_____

4) _____

_____

5) _____

_____

6) _____

_____

Identify potential accountability partners. A good accountability partner for me would be:

1) _____

2) _____

3) _____

If you do not have someone in your life that you feel would make a good accountability partner, try reaching out to local or online support groups. Support groups such as SAA, SA or Virtuous Pedophiles may be good places to find positive mentors and accountability partners in your community.

Impact and Consequences

A note about the consequences to others: your CSEM use impacts other people in your life. Your CSEM use also impacts the victims of these images. Remember the impact on the victims, how these images were created and the lack of control that victims have on the accessibility of their images circulating online. Remember the negative impact that CSEM use had on you. Taking the time to remember consequences is part of ensuring a healthy and offense free life.

The victims in the CSEM images matter.

These victims did not choose to have you watch them.

The children may have been exploited, tricked or manipulated.

Sexual images may have been stolen and uploaded online.

Some victims were simply too young to be able to make decisions about their sexual well-being.

Victims did not have any choice in <u>your</u> use of their image.

These are children.

Consider the impact of your actions on others to help keep you accountable. Whether that negative consequence involves you, others in your life or the victims in the CSEM images, child exploitation harms us all!

One consequence of your use of CSEM is that you have likely lost the trust of your friends and loved ones. If you were involved in the criminal justice system, you have lost the trust of your community. You may also feel that you have lost trust in yourself and your own ability to make good choices. Regaining trust takes much more time than it takes to lose trust. <u>Building trust is possible, but it takes time</u>.

If you want to rebuild trust in your relationships, you will need to demonstrate your ability to make good choices. You may have to give people the ability to monitor your behaviors in much more detail. It is not unusual for partners, friends and/or loved ones to want firm proof that you are making good decisions. They may treat all your decisions with suspicion. They may want to track your whereabouts. They may surprise you at different times or at different places (for example, at work or during leisure activities) to make sure that you are doing what you said you would be doing. They may want to read all your online communications and verify your online activities. They may not want you to access computers in a private space. People who are in your life may want to receive accountability reports from your Internet monitoring software. Provide them with the reassurance that they seek. They are likely afraid to trust you. Offer them safety.

Does it make you angry when people want proof that you are making good choices?

If so, examine what is making you angry. Is your reaction warranted? How will your anger impact this relationship? It can help to ask yourself, "What fear, anxiety or concern is motivating those who are seeking reassurance?"

The best strategy to rebuild trust is to openly accept scrutiny. If you are making the right choices, scrutiny is fine. If you find that you react badly to scrutiny, then maybe you are not being honest with yourself or with others about your decisions, your intentions or your choices. Alternatively, maybe you are again focusing too much on your wants and desires instead of the needs of those around you. By offering your loved ones safety, you may start slowly to rebuild trust. Consider asking your family, friends and loved ones what they need to feel safe.

Breaches of trust worsen if there already has been a breach of trust in the relationship. A second breach of trust can be very difficult to repair. If you have breached trust in the past, it will be difficult for loved ones to accept your assurances. If you continue to breach trust, their ability to trust you will erode. In other words, you can rebuild trust once if you are open and honest about your behaviors. Should you continue to break promises, lie about your activities and/or are deceitful in any way, rebuilding trust in your relationships will no longer be an option. You will lose the relationship.

What do my family, friends or loved ones need to feel safe?

1) _____

_____

2) _____

_____

3) _____

_____

4) _____

_____

5) _____

_____

6) _____

_____

7) _____

_____

8) _____

_____

Do I want to provide safety to my loved ones? Why or why not?

_____

_____

_____

_____

_____

_____

Partners, families and loved ones likely will struggle with your past choices. Learning that you have committed a crime that involves children and sexuality can be extremely difficult for others in your life to understand and/or accept. They suffer multiple losses as a result of your actions. Losing trust in someone is a loss. It is a loss to learn that you have been deceived. It is a loss to learn that someone you love has committed a crime. There may be other losses, such as the involvement of criminal justice authorities and/or child protection services.

Being there for your loved ones requires you to be able to truly acknowledge your mistake. It also requires a firm guarantee that you will better manage your behavior in the future. Genuine apologies are one important step in this process.

To complete a genuine apology, you must acknowledge that what you did was wrong and take full responsibility for causing harm to others. It is often helpful to explain your understanding about why you accessed CSEM and outline your specific plan to avoid any similar behaviors in the future. It is a good idea when you are apologizing to demonstrate regret for your actions. Being able to show that you truly understand and care about the negative consequences that others have suffered because of your actions is an essential component of a genuine apology. Finally, you may want to offer a way to repair the situation or something that you can do in order to truly demonstrate your understanding of the gravity of your actions. A genuine apology requires you to be truly sorry. An apology does not equal forgiveness. Often people engage in apology with the expectation that they will be forgiven. That is not a helpful apology; that is a self-centered apology. People will choose whether they will forgive you for your actions. They are not required to do so, and they may never do so. A genuine apology acknowledges harm and responsibility for having done harm. It can be a first step in rebuilding relationships and helping others heal.

Another important step when you are communicating with loved ones is to clearly explain themes related to longstanding vulnerabilities, triggers and the content of your self-management plan. Simply telling them not to worry won't help. You must give them detailed information that allows them to understand how your use of CSEM happened. This will allow them to better comprehend behaviors that are likely very difficult for them to understand.

The changes that you make as a result of your safety plan should be noticeable by your loved ones. They should be able to notice specific changes in your behaviors, new thinking patterns and new ways that you manage your emotions. Your loved ones should be encouraged to identify both positive changes and areas of concern that they observe. Hopefully you have included your loved ones in your work throughout these chapters. If not, you can review your work with them now.

Loved ones seek understanding. This understanding comes from full disclosure. Being honest with your loved ones will help set the foundation for the building of trust. Find a time where you can be uninterrupted to speak with your loved ones. Explain what happened. Understand that by discussing your CSEM use with others, they may choose to end their relationships with you. That can be a frightening possibility; however, if the relationship is truly important to you, how can that relationship be healthy and respectful if you are not honest? Giving people information provides them with the respect they need to form a more positive relationship with you in the future – should they choose to.

Due to the negative impact of your CSEM use on your loved ones, expect that they will need to focus on their own self-care during this time. Encouraging loved ones to take the time to address their needs, exercise, make healthy food choices and talk with a trusted friend or therapist can be helpful.

You may want to seek couples counseling, family counseling and/or additional individual counseling to assist you in your efforts to rebuild positive relationships with your loved ones.

In conclusion, there are many ways to ensure accountability in your life. This involves acknowledging the responsibility that you have toward other people in your life. Finding mentors, friends, partners and/or other support people with whom to share your journey is important. Open communication is a powerful key to addressing the myriad negative consequences that your loved ones have experienced as a result of your actions. Providing relevant information and a genuine apology can be a first step. Relationships with loved ones may end and you may need to grieve those losses. If your loved ones choose to rebuild a trusting relationship with you, ensure that you are willing to face scrutiny and make choices that will confirm their trust in you. This journey is completed in many small steps; rebuilding trust takes time.

CHAPTER SUMMARY

- Ask for help! Create an accountability team to assist you with applying and maintaining your safety plan
- There are many negative consequences that occur as a result of your prior use of CSEM
- Your loved ones are impacted by your behaviors
- You will have to rebuild trust following your viewing of CSEM
- Building trust will take time
- Genuine apologies along with relevant information about your longstanding vulnerabilities, triggers and safety plan may help
- Work cooperatively with your loved ones so that they feel safe
- Seek the help of a couples counselor and/or attend workshops for couples for additional assistance to rebuild trust in your spousal relationship. For other relationships, work with your individual therapist to help rebuild trust in your relationships.

14

Concluding Comments

CLINICIAN GUIDE

At this point, you have worked through the entire treatment plan. The client has completed the chapters aimed at ceasing and managing their use of CSEM. Throughout these chapters, the building of trust, therapeutic alliance and creating positive successes for the client have been key.

Maintenance sessions occur once the treatment plan is completed. These sessions are focused on helping the client maintain their gains and address any risks that may occur. It also allows the client to receive support as they continue to manage longstanding vulnerabilities. Encouraging the client to participate in group or individual maintenance programs is a good way to maintain their gains over time.

At the end of this workbook, if the client is managing well, you may or may not recommend ongoing maintenance sessions. It is our recommendation that maintenance sessions are generally helpful and can provide accountability to clients. It will be important for you as a clinician in collaboration with the client to decide what will be in your client's best interests. We encourage you to ensure that the client has a plan to review and adjust their safety plan over time. The safety plan continues to be a live document that is expected to change and shift with the client's changing life circumstances.

As you complete the treatment plan, help the client celebrate their gains and reward their hard work. As a clinician, focus on the positive changes you have observed within the client and communicate these changes clearly to them. You may also want to highlight some areas of continued difficulty that you would like them to monitor moving forward. Discuss ways to integrate rewards to help motivate the client in their continued work toward their goals. Learning to reward themselves for their successes, their goals achieved and/or their progress made toward their goals is an important element for maintaining change.

Clinicians are encouraged to assist the client to practice their skills and to build on their current successes in order to address outstanding issues. Often, the client is willing to explore and improve their functioning in other areas of their lives once they have completed this work and improved their understanding of their personal dynamics. Additional topics of exploration could include issues such as childhood sexual abuse, couples counseling, sexual therapy and/or other related topics. You may also want to provide the client with recommended readings to explore issues that require ongoing reflection. There is a list of our recommended readings by subject located at the end of this workbook. Remember that some

DOI: 10.4324/9781003388142-15

clients will prefer audiobooks rather than written material. Most books are currently available in both print and audio versions.

In conclusion, we hope that you have found this workbook to be helpful to you. As a mental health practitioner, we expect that you will find working with this client group just as exciting, interesting and fulfilling as we do. Good luck in your clinical journey — we wish you all the best!

CLIENT WORKBOOK

In conclusion, we hope that this journey has been positive and helpful for you. It took courage to start this journey, and your hard work has brought much progress. We trust that you have made changes to your life, your relationships, your thinking patterns, your emotions management, your sexuality and your computer use. These changes are important in helping you achieve your good life. We hope that you continue to strive to make your life work for you, while managing any illegal thoughts or illegal activities. Celebrate your successes and keep working at maintaining the progress you have made.

Celebrating success means that you build in positive rewards for making the changes to your life that keep you and others safe. What healthy rewards would be meaningful to you? Finding ways to acknowledge your efforts and your changes can be a powerful motivator. Don't be afraid to reward yourself for the positive changes you have made. Do you want to give yourself small incentives for having a good week or a good month? Or would you rather build in a more substantial reward for great changes over the next year? Acknowledging your success will be helpful to you.

Maintaining your efforts is the key to success. Maintenance is what keeps you from slipping. Maintenance keeps you focused on your goals. Maintenance allows you to continue making good choices. You engage in maintenance when you review these materials regularly, when you check in both with yourself and with your accountability partners about your progress and when you check on how you are applying your safety plan. Take the time to review your safety plan on a regular basis.

Maintenance matters. You may engage in maintenance by working productively with a group of people in the community who are working on the same goals, or you may engage in maintenance on your own. Remember to reach out for additional help if you need it.

Finding satisfaction in your life can sometimes occur with the smallest of steps. Making positive changes can help you stay on track and begin to truly enjoy your life again. You are encouraged to continue your journey, one step at a time! Good luck!

Recommended Readings

If you don't like to read, most of these books are available as audio books as well!

Attention Deficit Hyperactivity Disorder

Hallowell, E. M., & Ratey, J. J. (2021). *ADHD 2.0: New science and essential strategies for striving without distraction from childhood through adulthood*. New York: Random House Publishing Group.

Hiscock, H., & Sciberras, E. (Eds.). (2019). *Sleep and ADHD: An evidence-based guide to assessment and treatment*. San Diego, CA: Academic Press.

Orlov, M. (2010). *The ADHD effect on marriage: Understand and rebuild your relationship in six steps*. Plantation, FL: Speciality Press/A.D.D. Warehouse.

Vincent, A. (2017). *My brain still needs glasses*. Irvine, CA: Juniper Publishing.

Anger Management

Cullen, M., & Freeman-Longo, R. E. (1996). *Men & anger: Understanding and managing your anger for a much better life*. Holyoke, MA: NEARI Press.

Harbin, T. J. (2018). *Beyond anger: A guide for men: How to free yourself from the grip of anger and get more out of life*. Cambridge, MA: Da Capo Press.

Moes, M., & Proaño, A. (2016). *Lose your temper: A conscious exploration of anger*. Vancouver, BC: Moose Anger Management.

Schiraldi, G. R., & Kerr, M. H. (2002). *The anger management sourcebook*. New York: Contemporary Books.

Anxiety and Depression – Mood Disorders

Bourne, E. J. (2015). *The anxiety & phobia workbook*. Oakland, CA: New Harbinger Publications.

Burns, D. D. (1981). *Feeling good: The new mood therapy*. New York, NY: Penguin Books.

Dow, M. (2015). *The brain fog fix*. New York: Hay House, Inc.

Greenberger, D., & Padesky, C. A. (2016). *Mind over mood: Change how you feel by changing the way you think* (2nd ed.). New York: Guildford Press.

Hanson, R., & Mendius, R. (2009). *Buddha's brain: The practical neuroscience of happiness, love & wisdom*. Oakland, CA: New Harbinger Publications.

Hayes, S. C. (2005). *Get out of your mind & into your life*. Oakland, CA: New Harbinger Publications.

Jeffers, S. J. (1988). *Feel the fear and do it anyway*. New York: Ballantine.

Paterson, R. J. (2016). *How to be miserable*. Oakland, CA: New Harbinger Publications.

Paterson, R. J. (2020). *How to be miserable in your twenties: 40 ways to fail at adulting*. New Oakland, CA: Harbinger Publications.

Pittman, C. M., & Karle, E. M. (2015). *Rewire your anxious brain: How to use the neuroscience of fear to end anxiety, panic, and worry*. Oakland, CA: New Harbinger Publications.

DOI: 10.4324/9781003388142-16

Siegel, D. (2018). *Aware: The science and practice of presence – The groundbreaking meditation practice*. New York: TarcherPerigee.

Wehrenberg, M. (2008). *The 10 best-ever anxiety management techniques: Understanding how your brain makes you anxious & what you can do to change it*. New York: W.W. Norton Company.

Childhood Abuse

Levine, P. A. (2010). *In an unspoken voice. How the body releases trauma and restores goodness*. Berkeley, CA: North Atlantic Books.

Singer, K. (2010). *Evicting the perpetrator: A male survivor's guide for recovery from childhood sexual abuse*. Holyoke, MA: NEARI Press.

Van der Kolk, B. A. (2015). *The body keeps the score: Brain, mind, and body in the healing of trauma*. New York: Penguin Books.

Walker, P. (2013). *Complex PTSD: From surviving to thriving*. Lafayette, CA: Azure Coyote Publishing.

Pain Management

Caudill, M., & Herbert, B. (2016). *Managing pain before it manages you*. New York: The Guilford Press.

Gordon, A. (2020). *The way out: A revolutionary, scientifically proven approach to healing chronic pain*. New York: Avery Publications.

Relationships and General Wellness

Ansari, A., & Klinenberg, E. (2015). *Modern romance*. New York: Penguin Press.

Brown, B. (2008). *I thought it was just me (but it isn't): Telling the truth about perfectionism, inadequacy, and power*. New York: Gotham Books.

Brown, B. (2012). *Daring greatly: How the courage to be vulnerable transforms the way we live, love, parent, and lead*. New York: Avery.

Brown, B. (2015). *Rising strong* (1st ed.). New York: Spiegel & Grau.

Brown, B. (2017). *Braving the wilderness: The quest for true belonging and the courage to stand alone*. New York: Random House.

Brown, B. (2018). *Dare to lead: Brave work. Tough conversations. Whole hearts*. New York: Random House.

Browne, J. (2011). *Dating for dummies*. Hoboken, NJ: For Dummies Publications.

Gottman, J. M., & Silver, N. (2015). *The seven principles for making marriage work*. New York: Harmony Press.

Gottman, J. M., & Schwartz Gottman, J. (2022). *The love prescription*. London: Penguin Books.

Gottman, J. M., Schwartz Gottman, J., Abrams, D., & Carlton Abrams, R. (2016). *The man's guide to women: Scientifically proven secrets from the "Love Lab" about what women really want*. Emmaus, PA: Rodale Books.

Gottman, J. M., Schwartz Gottman, J., Abrams, D., & Carleton Abrams, J. (2019). *Eight dates: Essential conversations for a lifetime of love*. New York: Workman Publishing Company.

Harper, F. G. (2020). *Unf#ck your boundaries workbook: Build better relationships through consent, communication, and expressing your needs*. Microcosm Publishing.

Levine, A., & Heller, R. S. F. (2011). *Attached: The new science of adult attachment and how it can help you find – and keep – love*. New York: TarcherPerigee.

Paterson, R. J. (2000). *The assertiveness workbook: How to express your ideas and stand up for yourself at work and in relationships*. Oakland, CA: New Harbinger Publications.

Wachs, K. M. (2002). *Relationships for dummies*. Hoboken, NJ: For Dummies Publications.

Weiss, R. (2017). *Out of the doghouse: A step-by-step relationship-saving guide for men caught cheating*. Deerfield Beach, FL: Health Communications, Inc.

Young, J. E., & Klosko, J. S. (1994). *Reinventing your life: The breakthrough program to end negative behavior . . . and feel great again*. New York: Plume.

Sexuality

Kerner, I. (2010). *She comes first: The thinking man's guide to pleasuring a woman*. New York, NY: Harper Collins Publications.

Langford, J. (2016). *Spare me "the talk"!: A girl's guide to sex, relationships, and growing up*. Mercer Island, WA: ParentMap.

Langford, J. (2019). *Spare me "the talk"!: A guy's guide to sex, relationships, and growing up*. Mercer Island, WA: ParentMap.

McCarthy, B. W., & Metz, M. E. (2004). *Coping with premature ejaculation: How to overcome PE, please your partner and have great sex*. Oakland, CA: New Harbinger Publications.

Metz, M. E., & McCarthy, B. W. (2004). *Coping with erectile dysfunction: How to regain confidence and enjoy great sex*. Oakland, CA: New Harbinger Publications.

Westheimer, R. K., & Lehu, P. A. (2019). *Sex for dummies* (4th ed.). Hoboken, NJ: Wiley & Sons.

Sleep Hygiene

Hauri, P., & Linde, S. M. (1996). *No more sleepless nights*. New York: Wiley.

Hiscock, H., & Sciberras, E. (2019). *Sleep and ADHD: An evidence-based guide to assessment and treatment*. San Diego, CA: Academic Press.

Author Biographies

Dr. Lyne Piché, Ph.D. Lyne is a registered psychologist who has worked in the field of Forensic Psychology for 25 years. She has worked in both federal and provincial correctional settings. She received her doctorate degree from the Université du Québec à Montréal in 1998, specializing in clinical and research psychology. Her studies focused on assessing and treating sexual dysfunctions and paraphilias. Since 1998, she has provided both assessment and treatment services for men who have committed violent and sexual offenses. Lyne has given presentations related to sexuality, intimacy, sexual offending and risk assessment throughout her career. She is regularly invited to present workshops on issues related to the assessment and treatment of men who access child sexual exploitation material. She has published on the topic of sexuality and sexual offending. Throughout her career, she has worked with many clients of differing cultures and backgrounds. She enjoys working with adults, youths and people with special needs. She particularly enjoys teaching students who are new to the field. In addition, Lyne is an EMDRIA certified EMDR therapist for trauma therapy. In her practice, she focuses on improving sexual health, understanding neurodiversity and exploring all types of relationships.

Dr. Anton Schweighofer, R. Psych. Anton is a registered psychologist who received his doctorate in clinical psychology from Simon Fraser University in Vancouver, Canada, in 1998. His primary areas of interest have included forensic psychology and addictions. Anton was employed with the Correctional Service of Canada (CSC) for over ten years; prior to leaving the Correctional Service of Canada in 2009, he was the Senior Psychologist for sex offense-specific programming, and he also acted as the regional Chief of Psychology (Pacific Region). Anton has maintained a private practice that has included forensic risk assessment and treatment since 2000. He has given presentations on sex offense issues and risk assessment at national and international conferences. He is regularly invited to present a pre-conference workshop for the Association for the Treatment and Prevention of Sexual Abuse (ATSA) conference on issues related to the assessment and treatment of men who access child sexual exploitation material. He is a national trainer for the Static-99R, which is the most widely used actuarial measure for estimating risk for sexual reoffense. He has provided expert testimony to the courts with regard to sex offense issues, the use of risk measures with Indigenous offenders and is among those designated to provide Dangerous Offender assessments as an amicus curiae. Finally, he is a 23-year member of ATSA, an ATSA Fellow, and served as the co-chairperson at the 2011 ATSA conference.

Index

Note: Page numbers in *italic* indicate a figure on the corresponding page.